ADDICTION TO PRESCRIPTION PAIN KILLERS AND THE STREET DRUG HEROIN

A GUIDE TO UNDERSTANDING AND OVERCOMING OPIOID DEPENDENCY AND OPIOID ADDICTION

GREGORY H. PIERCE M.D.

ISBN: 0-615-51207-0
ISBN-13: 978-0-615-51207-5

I dedicate this book to the countless patients whom I have had the pleasure of serving and who have faithfully entrusted their care to me. I am also grateful for my lovely wife, Sherie. She has worked by my side as an addiction counselor and has been instrumental in helping me reach my goals.

CONTENTS

About the Author, and the Goal of the Book.................................i

Acknowledgements vii

CHAPTER 1:
The Opioid Drug Problem In America 1

CHAPTER 2:
The History of Opioids and Their Definition............................ 5

CHAPTER 3:
How Do Opioids Work? 15

CHAPTER 4:
Why Do People Misuse Opioids and Develop Addictions? 21

CHAPTER 5:
Opioid Dependency... 25

CHAPTER 6:
Opioid Addiction 27

CHAPTER 7:
Is Opioid Addiction a Disease? 31

CHAPTER 8:
Treatments for Opioid Dependency and Addiction 35

CHAPTER 9:
Seeds for Success 59

CHAPTER 10:
Managing Withdrawal 71

CHAPTER 11:
Conclusion 77

References 81

ABOUT THE AUTHOR, AND THE GOAL OF THE BOOK

I have had the privilege and pleasure of practicing medicine in Philadelphia and Montgomery counties, in Pennsylvania, for the past thirty years. During these years, much of my time has been spent helping people with substance abuse problems and addictive behaviors. Early in my medical practice, I participated in a five-year residency at Temple University Hospital in Philadelphia, Pennsylvania, and I was the chief surgical resident in the general and trauma surgery department for the last two years of my residency. It was very challenging, with a lot of late hours spent doing emergency surgeries for stab wound and gunshot victims. I learned how to determine what was wrong and how to perform complicated surgical procedures under very stressful conditions. Even in the most chaotic and challenging situations, I learned to be calm, remain confident in my capabilities, and persevere until the task was completed.

Upon completion of my training, I went into private practice and began specializing in the treatment of patients with eating disorders. I was performing bariatric surgery and vertical banded gastroplasty, and was providing the endoscopic placement of a device called the "gastric bubble," for morbidly obese patients. It was during this experience that I became interested in the counseling and nutritional components of treating morbid obesity. I also noticed that the overwhelming majority of these patients were suffering from low self-esteem and poor body images. No matter how much weight they lost, when they looked at themselves in the mirror, they still saw an obese person. I believed these negative feelings and emotions encouraged the continuation of the maladaptive behaviors and poor eating habits that contributed to their being morbidly obese. It became apparent to me that without a patient's awareness and understanding of the nature of his or her problem, and of the necessity for behavior modification, an eating disorder could not be fully corrected. As a motivational tool and as part of patients' treatment, I started doing cosmetic surgery procedures to surgically remove the excess fat and sagging skin, and rejuvenate their bodies.

My father, Harold E. Pierce Jr., MD, was a renowned dermatologist and a pioneer in the field of cosmetic surgery. He and I worked side-by-side in the same office, and he was responsible for my gaining the surgical skills and judgment required to perform these cosmetic procedures. It was my belief that by reconstructing and visually enhancing the bodies of the morbidly obese patients this would significantly improve how they felt about themselves. With a more positive outlook and mood, they would be motivated to make better decisions regarding eating habits and would put more effort into their physical conditioning programs. The resulting behavioral changes would then ultimately ensure a better outcome, with more lasting results. I spent close to fifteen years working in the field of cosmetic surgery.

Throughout my career in medicine, I always wanted to help people overcome obstacles and make a significant difference in their lives. My personal relationship with God helped me overcome many challenges and as I grew spiritually, I was called to become an ordained minister in a Christian church. My ministry revolved around motivating and teaching people how to overcome the many obstacles confronting them in their daily lives. I primarily worked with homeless and disenfranchised individuals who oftentimes were battling substance abuse and addictions. I supported their efforts with food, shelter, job placement, and spiritual guidance. I also took the time to fellowship with them because there is no better way to show that you truly care about someone than to share a part of your life with him or her. The connection made between two people when one empathizes with another's predicament, believes in the person, and does not stand in judgment can be a motivating force for changing that person's behavior. As I became more involved with the fight against illicit drug use, I noticed how drug abuse was destroying certain neighborhoods in the inner city of Philadelphia. I became a member of the Philadelphia Police Clergy, and together with other clergy and church members, we targeted drug-infested street corners in Philadelphia. We identified the street corners where open drug dealing was ongoing, and flagrantly and physically, as a large group, took over the drug corner. Through these spirited encounters, I also had the pleasure of working with another organization called Mothers Against Drugs (MAD). Together we handed out pamphlets encouraging drug users to seek treatment, and we stopped any drug exchanges from taking place. I learned many valuable lessons from these experiences, and what stood out was this: In order to lead people and help them change their lives for the better, you need to be humble, tolerant, strong, and courageous, and, above all, lead by example.

When I became a Certified Personal Trainer for the National Strength and Conditioning Association, I greatly expanded on my ability to treat eating disorders and addictive behaviors. Part of my training was focused on studying nutrition and herbology, and I became proficient at developing specialized meal plans. I also incorporated my personal experiences from training in tai chi, and my expertise as a second-degree black belt in Shotokan karate, to create comprehensive exercise programs. Interestingly enough, what I found to be most challenging was motivating and inspiring people to commit to making the necessary lifestyle and behavioral changes necessary to successfully reach their goals. What made a big difference, and what allowed me to be successful at this, was my ability to understand what their obstacles to change were, to communicate cogently to them, and relate to them effectively. I also participated in physically rehabilitating people who were suffering from physical injuries, disabilities, and debilitating diseases. A lot of those people had chronic pain, and this lead me to become educated and certified as a pain management specialist by the American Academy of Pain Management. Since drug abuse, drug dependence, and drug addiction in chronic pain patients ranges between 3 and 19 percent (Fishbain, 1992), I decided to get the training so I could be licensed by the Drug Enforcement Agency to prescribe Suboxone. Suboxone is the only medication that can be prescribed in a private doctor's office for the treatment of prescription painkiller and heroin dependencies and addictions. A dependency means the drug user can function normally as long as the drug is in their system, whereas with an addiction the user cannot function normally regardless. For the past six years of my medical practice, I have specialized exclusively with treatment for prescription painkiller and heroin dependencies and addictions, and for pain management. After I became board certified by the American Board of Addiction Medicine, I was appointed the medical director of two methadone clinics. Methadone therapy programs have historically served as the gold standard for the treatment of patients who have addictions to prescription painkillers and heroin. My skills as a physician, teacher, personal trainer, martial artist, and minister, along with my life experiences, have allowed me to function as a life coach for my patients. I enjoy helping them identify their goals and the obstacles to reaching those goals. I inspire them to make the necessary changes to be successful to reach their goals, and help them find joy and a sense of accomplishment in their lives.

In performing my life's work, I have personally witnessed not only the devastation that painkiller and heroin addictions can have on my patients' lives, but also the tragic rippling effect it has on the lives of their families and loved ones. Families, neighborhoods, and extended communities have suffered financial and spiritual bankruptcy because of this plague. These experiences in what have now become my passion and my profession have inspired me to write this book, so that I could help the individuals and the families affected by this complicated problem. It has been my experience that the public and the majority of the medical community lack a basic understanding of this affliction. When confronted with people who are dependent on narcotic painkillers and heroin, they respond with fear, anger, frustration, and ridicule. This reaction then fosters in the dependent and addicted individual's feelings of hopelessness, defeatism, and self-loathing. Family members and loved ones become confused and feel betrayed and powerlessness over the situation.

By reading this book, your questions will be answered, and you will be given the information and understanding you need to develop an effective strategy to overcome and fix this complicated problem. Understanding the nature of this condition and how it happens is akin to laying down fertile soil, which will serve as our foundation. You will also be given sixteen seeds that, when planted in this enriched soil, will blossom and bear a prosperous and fulfilled life free from attachments to habit-forming and addictive drugs. I like to call this process *evolutionary therapy*. It requires varying degrees of self-navigation, depending on the severity and nature of the problem, and will ultimately lead to constructive self-management of one's life. I have never met a single person who asked for, or wanted to have, a chemical dependency or addiction. But those who are afflicted can decide to get better. The moment people make that decision, they have taken the most important step and have already started their recovery. With the proper help and guidance, they can be an even better person than before.

ACKNOWLEDGMENTS

I am grateful for the grace of God and anointing of the Holy Spirit, through the acceptance of Jesus Christ as my Lord and Savior, without which this undertaking and its completion would not have been possible.

CHAPTER 1

THE OPIOID DRUG PROBLEM IN AMERICA

To say that in the United States we have a problem with prescription painkiller and heroin use is an understatement. No one would argue that over the past ten to fifteen years, prescription painkiller use and abuse has increased at an alarming rate. The 2006 National Survey on Drug Use and Health by the Department of Health and Human Services gave us frightening statistics. For Americans aged twelve and older, the number of people who had abused painkillers in the month prior to being surveyed had increased from 2.6 million in 1999 to 5.2 million in 2006. Of that 5.2 million, 2.2 million were first-time users, which were higher than any other abused drug, including the number of first-time marijuana users. Painkiller abuse has become an epidemic in America and is, I believe, indicative of a much larger problem. Americans rely too heavily on chemicals to adjust their mood, enhance their daily performance, and escape the problems in their lives. The compulsive use, ingestion of, and overreliance on caffeinated products, tobacco, alcohol, junk food, prescription medication, and illegal drugs is contributing to an array of chronic diseases and conditions that threaten our society's very survival. Heart disease and cancer, which are the leading two causes of death in America, along with diabetes and mental health diseases, are directly linked to these compulsive and addictive behaviors. What's even more alarming is that when the National Survey on Drug Use and Health asked the people abusing painkillers where they were getting the drugs, roughly 60 percent of the respondents stated that they got their narcotic painkillers from a friend or relative, and 15 percent said they stole the drug from a friend or relative. This means that a significant portion of the American public is knowingly or unknowingly engaging in risky and illegal behavior without considering and acknowledging the harm it can produce. As long as there is no transfer of money involved, many people don't believe that they are committing a crime by giving a friend or a family member a controlled substance. The truth is that just by giving a narcotic drug prescribed to one person to another individual; these people are committing a felony and the crime of drug trafficking, and can be punished under our penal code system. They probably aren't even considering the possible side effects, drug interactions, and potential lethal complications that can occur, and are ignorant of the message this behavior sends to our youth. People need to understand that the laws and rules are there not to just protect us from other people, but also to protect us from ourselves. Twenty percent of the respondents obtained their narcotic painkillers from a doctor's office. Doctors who prescribe narcotic painkillers have to make sure that there is a clear indication and need for the medication, and that the benefit from prescribing it outweighs the risk of taking it. Doctors should also educate their patients on the risk of developing a chemical dependency or addiction, and make certain that they store the medication safely, so the potential of accidental poisoning and theft are minimized. Doctors should call patients in for random pill counts and perform random urine drug testing, and be aware of the signs that a patient may be misusing his or her medication and/or diverting it by either giving it to a friend or selling it on the street.

What I have found helpful in my practice is not to accept any patient referrals or walk-ins for pain management. I make sure all of my referrals come from a professional in the field with the appropriate and supporting medical records. After I review that material, I make the decision as to whether or not the prospective patient should be scheduled for an evaluation to see if he or she meets the criteria for specialized pain management. The fact that in the National Survey on Drug Use and Health only 4 percent of the respondents received their narcotic painkiller from a drug dealer, and less than 1 percent from the Internet, shows us that the problem is not what most people might have expected. Heroin is a dangerous and highly addictive drug, and its usage has also increased. To partially account for underestimation of heroin use due to under reporting, an adjustment based on counts of arrest and clients in treatment has been applied to the National Household Survey on Drug Abuse data, resulting in estimates of 2.9 million lifetime users and 663 thousand past year users (National Drug Control Strategy, 1996). The temptations for using heroin compared to the narcotic painkillers are that it can cost less to use, initially, and it provides a greater reward, or high. Of course, when the user becomes addicted, he or she invariably ends up spending more money, exhibiting more dysfunctional behaviors, and has the added risk of contracting infectious hepatitis, HIV, and endocarditis (infection of the heart valves).

CHAPTER 2

THE HISTORY OF OPIOIDS
AND THEIR DEFINITION

Let's take a lesson in history and, in the process, get rid of any confusion that may exist among words like *drugs, painkillers, heroin,* and *narcotics.* **A drug is any substance that, when introduced into the body, changes how the body works.** Opium is a drug that numbs the senses and creates a euphoric dreamlike state. It is one of the oldest drugs known to humankind, and its use dates back to 5,000 B.C. It is obtained from the poppy plant and was used in the ancient Egyptian, Greek, and Roman empires for food, as an anesthetic to relieve pain, by soldiers to dull their senses to danger, and for religious rituals (Aggrawal, 1995). Its recreational use became popular in China around the early 1600s, and by the late 1700s it was being imported by Britain into China, where addictions to opium had become prevalent (SACU, 2006). Around the early 1800s, the chemical morphine was extracted from opium by a German pharmacologist and was manufactured and marketed as a safe alternative to opium. However, morphine, like opium, not only relieved pain but also created an extremely pleasurable dreamlike state, which made it quite habit forming. In the

1850s during the California Gold Rush, thousands of Americans, Latin Americans, Europeans, Australians, and Chinese migrated to California. Opium dens were established in the western states of America and became popular destinations for rest, relaxation, and entertainment. When the American Civil War began in 1861, the soldiers fighting in the war sustained a high number of traumatic injuries that required amputations and other surgical procedures. Morphine, which had been marketed as an anesthetic and pain reliever, was readily available and used extensively. Consequently, thousands of soldiers ended up using morphine on a regular basis. In the late 1800s, a chemist in England developed a new chemical called diacetylmorphine, which was created from morphine. It was eventually trademarked as "Heroin" in Germany, so it could be manufactured and marketed as a safe alternative to morphine and could be used in the treatment of morphine addictions. Drug companies began purchasing habit-forming drugs like heroin, morphine, and cocaine, and selling them directly to the public. They packaged them as tonics and elixirs containing one or more of these drugs, or individually, with a needle and syringe. These drugs became available in drugstores in America and were marketed as cures for both physical and mental ailments, such as cancer, arthritis, depression, fatigue, coughs, and colds. Doctors were also prescribing these drugs liberally in their medical practices. What ensued was a major morphine, heroin, and opium epidemic in America. These practices didn't stop until 1914, when the United States Congress enacted legislation through the Harrison Narcotics Tax Act. This act required doctors and pharmacists who prescribed narcotics to register and pay a tax. After the creation of the U.S. Treasury Department's Narcotics Division—the first federal drug agency—habit-forming drugs that posed significant health risk and danger to our society were either outlawed or had access to them limited. It was determined that heroin and opium could not be used safely for any purpose, and they were outlawed, while morphine and cocaine use was restricted. Unfortunately, hundreds of thousands of individuals addicted to these drugs were now vulnerable to illicit drug dealers and in desperate need of treatment. As the problem of illicit drug use and drug addiction continued to progress in America, Congress made the decision in 1973 to coordinate all the federal government's drug control efforts in the hope they would be more effective against the growing drug problem. To accomplish this, they combined the different entities under one agency, called the Drug Enforcement Agency, or DEA. As the fight against illicit and dangerous drugs waged on, the term "narcotic" came to mean a drug whose use is regulated and controlled by the federal government. Healthcare providers and chemists classify these narcotic drugs based on where they come from and how they work. Opium is a drug extracted from *papaver somniferum*, the poppy plant, which grows naturally. Any medication that relieves pain and is partly or completely derived from opium is called an "opiate." In the 1970s it was discovered that opium exerted its effect on the body by attaching to specific receptor sites. A receptor site is a docking port that allows chemicals and substances to land on tissues, and produces an effect on them. The receptor sites are located primarily in our bodies' central nervous system and gastrointestinal tracts, and the first one discovered was named the *mu-opioid* receptor site (Pert, 1973). There are four opioid receptor sites, named the *mu, kappa, delta* and *sigma* opioid receptor sites, with the *mu-opioid* being responsible for euphoria, pain relief, slowing of the heart rate, and respiratory depression, or difficulty breathing. Any chemical exerting its primary effect by binding to an opioid receptor site is classified an opioid. Codeine (found in Tylenol II, III, and IV) and morphine are extracted from the resin of the opium poppy and are examples of a naturally occurring opiate completely derived from opium. They fall into the broader class of opioids, because they work by binding to the opioid receptor sites. Heroin, oxycodone (Percocet and OxyContin), and hydrocodone (Vicodin, Lortab) are synthesized by humans, from opium or a derivative of opium, and are therefore also called opiates. Other painkillers, such as Fentanyl and methadone, are completely man-made and, consequently, are not opiates, but because they work by attaching to the opioid receptors, they *are* classified as opioids. Calling a drug a "narcotic" is more of a legal term, because it means the drug is either illegal or needs to be prescribed by a licensed doctor for a medical purpose. Prescription painkillers and heroin are called narcotics for legal reasons, and opioids because of how they work.

Another area of confusion is the generic name versus the brand name of a medication. A drug can either occur in nature or be engineered in a laboratory. When a pharmaceutical company researches and engineers a new chemical drug, it protects its investment by patenting the new drug. A patent affords the manufacturer of the new drug twenty years of protection from having another company produce and sell its drug. The manufacturer usually gives the drug a brand name for marketing purposes, and trademarks that name. This means that the manufacturer owns the name, and the product is protected against another company using that name, even after the patent on the drug expires. A "generic" drug is a drug that is produced and sold without a patent. Codeine, oxycodone, hydrocodone, morphine, and methadone are all examples of generic drugs with no patents on them. Tylenol is a trademarked brand name and is thereby owned by McNeal Consumer Healthcare, a subsidiary of Johnson & Johnson. The active ingredient and chemical drug in Tylenol is acetaminophen. When the patent for the drug named Tylenol expired, other companies were able to produce and sell acetaminophen as a generic drug, but they could not use the trademarked name "Tylenol." This is why you can go to the supermarket and buy Tylenol, or you can purchase acetaminophen, which is packaged and sold by a number of other companies. Either way, you are getting the same drug, and the generic form always costs less. Some people believe the companies that make the generic medications produce a less potent and effective drug and will insist on purchasing the more expensive brand name version of the drug. Tylenol II, III, and IV, which are combinations of acetaminophen and the narcotic opioid codeine, in varying strengths, are the trademarked brand names McNeal Consumer Healthcare uses to sell the drug it makes. Percocet is the trademarked brand name Endo Pharmaceuticals uses to sell its drug, which is a combination of acetaminophen and the narcotic opioid oxycodone. OxyContin ER is the trademarked brand name Purdue Pharma uses for its patented time-released formula of the narcotic opioid oxycodone. Vicodin is the trademarked brand name Abbot Laboratories uses for its drug, which is a combination of acetaminophen and the narcotic opioid hydrocodone. Fentanyl is the generic name for the trademarked drug Duragesic made by ALZA Corporation, whose patent has expired. Examples of commonly used generic narcotic opioids and their corresponding brand names are as follows:

Generic Drug	Trademarked Brand Name
Codeine and Acetaminophen	Tylenol II, II, IV
Morphine	MS Contin ER, Avinza ER, Kadian ER, Morphine Sulfate
Oxycodone	OxyContin ER, Oxy IR
Oxycodone and Acetaminophen	Percocet, Roxicet
Oxycodone and Aspirin	Percodan
Oxymorphone	Opana ER
Hydromorphone	Dilaudid
Hydrocodone	Tussionex (antitussive cough medicine)
Hydrocodone and Acetaminophen	Vicodin, Lorcet, Lortab, Vicoprofen, Norco
Buprenorphine	Subutex
Buprenorphine and Naloxone	Suboxone
Fentanyl	Duragesic, Fentora, Actiq

IR and ER stand for "instant release" and "extended release." The IR painkillers are instantly dissolved and absorbed in the gastrointestinal tract. The ER painkillers are coated with a special shell that delays their breakdown and absorption in the gastrointestinal tract and depending on the brand of ER tablet, its pain killing effect on the human body can last from twelve to twenty-four hours.

Whether the generic drugs, due to manufacturing practices, are less potent, and therefore less effective, has never been scientifically proven, but it is not uncommon for patients and healthcare providers to feel that they are, and insist on brand name only.

The human body makes its own opioids that attach to opioid receptors and are called endorphins. They are responsible for controlling our everyday aches and pains along with elevating our mood. When our bodies are faced with the challenge of relieving pain and managing stress, they will release endorphins that attach to the opioid receptor sites, which take awareness away from the pain and relieve stress. They are also released during exciting situations, and contribute to feelings of pleasure, including the feeling of love. Many physical therapy treatments and other measures used by doctors and physical therapists to manage pain partly work by assisting the human body in raising its own endorphin levels.

In summary, the opioids come from three different sources. They can grow in nature as the opium poppy plant, or be manufactured from a chemical derivative of that plant. They can be man-made and chemically engineered in a laboratory, or they can be made by the human body, in which case, they are referred to as endorphins. Possession and use of opioids found in nature or those that are man-made fall into a legal category and are called "narcotics," because they have to be prescribed by a doctor licensed by the DEA, and their use must be intended for medical purposes. Narcotic opioids which have been determined to be unsafe by the FDA, such as heroin, cannot be legally possessed or distributed in America, and are therefore illicit drugs.

Ironically, two man-made opioids have been found to be effective in treating the addictions that can arise from the use of opioids. One is methadone, which was developed and manufactured in Germany during World War II in the early 1940s. At that time, the Allied forces had been successful at establishing an embargo of Germany, which disrupted the flow of opium into the country. Some believe that in response a German scientist created Polamidon, which was later named "methadone," after the Allied forces seized all German patents at the conclusion of the war. However, it wasn't until after the war that methadone proved to be a very potent and effective painkiller whose effects lasted for over twenty-four hours (Chen, 1948). Until the mid-1960s, people with heroin addictions had little hope of living a normal life, because the heroin high only lasted for three to four hours and was followed by extremely painful and troubling withdrawal symptoms, called "dysphoria." These extreme highs and lows, and the erratic mood swings, produced the dysfunctional behavioral patterns seen with this addiction. Professor Emeritus Vincent Dole, his wife, and their colleagues started studying the effects of methadone in the treatment of heroin addictions at the Rockefeller University in New York. Their research showed methadone was able to remove cravings and withdrawals for at least twenty-four hours (Pate, 1997). The erratic highs and lows in mood associated with the euphoria, high, and dysphoria, were removed. As long as the patient took his or her methadone every twenty-four hours, he or she felt normal, didn't crave heroin, and was able to function normally (Pate, 1991).

The other opioid used in the treatment of opioid dependencies and addictions is buprenorphine. Buprenorphine is derived from thebaine, which is another substance that comes from the opium poppy plant. It was developed and manufactured by Reckitt Benckiser in the 1980s and trademarked as Temgesic for oral ingestion and Buprenex for intravenous use. These drugs were originally intended to be used as pain relievers during surgical procedures that required general anesthesia and marketed as such. Reckitt Benckiser renamed the buprenorphine and trademarked it as Subutex. During Reckitt Benckiser's research and attempt to gain FDA approval for the drug, the FDA had a major concern. It was afraid that abusers would crush up the Subutex and, instead of letting it dissolve under their tongue as intended, would inject it into their veins so they could get high from it. This would work particularly well if the person had never used opioids before. That's when the FDA decided to add a blocking drug, naloxone, which meant if the user had any opioids in his or her system and injected the Subutex, the abuser would go into immediate withdrawal and become violently ill. Reckitt Benckiser named the buprenorphine–naloxone combination Suboxone. The amount of naloxone in each Suboxone tablet is small enough not to be absorbed if placed under the tongue or accidently swallowed, but large enough to cause withdrawals if injected. Eventually, Reckitt Benckiser was successful in gaining FDA approval in 2002. Both Subutex and Suboxone were approved for detoxification and long-term management of opioid dependencies and addictions. Suboxone, Subutex, and methadone are similar in that they can prevent withdrawals and cravings without euphoria in the patient with an opioid addiction, which allows the patient to feel normal, become functional, and stop engaging in self-destructive and criminal behaviors.

Many steps and precautions have been taken in order to discourage the abuse and misuse of buprenorphine. Doctors have been instructed to primarily prescribe Suboxone, which contains the blocker naloxone. The only condition for using Subutex is if a patient is allergic to naloxone or is pregnant. In early 2011,

Reckitt Benckiser released the film delivery system for Suboxone. It was discovered that individuals who were chemically dependent on Suboxone were misusing and abusing it. Users would crush the pills and either inhale them nasally or inject them, and get high. In response the film was created, which cannot be crushed, inhaled, or injected. The film is also packaged in a container that has an individual serial number. When a patient receives his or her medication at the pharmacy, the corresponding number is recorded on a computer database. If the medication is diverted or sold, and ends up in police custody, it can be easily tracked back to the patient who purchased it at the pharmacy. If a doctor or a nurse is doing a pill count, detecting diversion is also easy because the serial numbers in each box of thirty films are individually coded and in sequential order. The generic form of Subutex—buprenorphine—became available in late 2009. The generic form of Suboxone—buprenorphine with naloxone—is not available yet because the manufacturers have been unable to duplicate the compound in a stable pill form.

Buprenorphine is still a good opioid painkiller and is thirty times more potent than morphine, but because buprenorphine is less active at the *mu*-opioid receptor, morphine is a stronger pain reliever, although buprenorphine has less cardiac and respiratory depression and chance of overdose. In July 2010, Purdue Pharma received FDA approval to market and sells its buprenorphine transdermal patch. This buprenorphine delivery system was trademarked as Butrans, and comes in three strengths. The patch is designed to stay on the skin for one week, and it is approved for the treatment of moderate to severe chronic pain.

CHAPTER 3

HOW DO OPIOIDS WORK?

Before discussing how opioids work, we must first have an understanding of how the brain works. Our brains are made up of nerve centers (neurons), communicating branches (axons), and chemicals (neurotransmitters). Think of it as resembling a circuit panel, or the motherboard of a computer. The neurons are connected to one another by the axons. Neurons are responsible for making and storing neurotransmitters. Neurons also have receptor sites seated on them, and each neurotransmitter has a specific receptor that it attaches to. The neurons communicate with one another by releasing the neurotransmitters, which attach to their receptors, which generates an electrical impulse that travels down the axon until it reaches another neuron. Every thought we have, every mood we experience, and every movement we make are the result of chemical reactions between the neurotransmitters and their receptors, which send an electrical impulse down the axon, communicating from cell to cell. When we put opioids in our bodies by chewing and/or swallowing, inhaling through our nostrils, or injecting them into our veins, they eventually get into our blood and become, or function as, neurotransmitters. When opioids reach the nervous tissues that make up our central nervous system, which includes our brain and spinal cord, they attach to any unoccupied opioid receptor site. This attachment causes a chemical reaction that dulls our senses and makes us pay little or no attention to the pain.

Neurotransmitters are chemicals that can be made by the human body or can be found naturally occurring in plants and other living creatures. Different neurotransmitters cause different chemical reactions and thereby different actions. We already know opioids relieve pain and improve our mood. Serotonin is a neurotransmitter that alters our mood and relieves depression. It is made in the human body's central nervous system and is found in certain foods such as cheese. Have you ever noticed when you feel depressed or overwhelmed, you have an urge to binge on ice cream, candy, or other type of sweets? This is your body trying to self- medicate your depression away. Sweets are primarily carbohydrates (sugar), and they cause our bodies to produce more serotonin, which relieves the depressed mood.

Our bodies make numerous neurotransmitters. The largest neurotransmitter mechanism in our bodies is the endocannabinoid system. This system is responsible for regulating pain sensation, mood, appetite, and numerous other bodily functions. The neurotransmitters that fuel this system are also found in marijuana. Much of the pharmaceutical companies' recent research is focused on developing new drugs that can regulate this system. Designer cannabinoids that mimic the effects of marijuana, when smoked, have also been manufactured and are sold in stores as K2 incense, Spice, and herbal incense. Since they are newly created chemicals, and in some instances haven't yet been scrutinized by the state and federal authorities, they are legal. They are very dangerous drugs that have been associated with signs of addiction (Zimmerman, 2009) and drug-induced psychosis (Muller, 2010).

On February 28, 2011, the DEA imposed an "emergency" ban to control the use of synthetic marijuana (Meserve, 2001).

Tobacco cigarettes contain a multitude of chemicals that can function as neurotransmitters and carcinogens (cancer-causing agents) in our bodies. Nicotine is a major ingredient found in cigarettes, and there are nicotine receptors in our central nervous system. When you smoke regularly, the number of nicotine receptors increases in your brain, and this contributes to the difficulty of quitting. The regulation of chemicals and neurotransmitters in our bodies is an important health consideration that we can control to varying degrees by choosing what we put into our bodies. Our choices dramatically influence our bodies' functioning from day to day, our length of life, and our quality of life.

Here is the interesting thing about opioids, which is the reason they are misused and why some people develop addictions: Not only do opioids attach to the opioid receptors and relieve pain, but they also cause a release of a neurotransmitter called "dopamine," in a particular area of our brain's mesolimbic system. The release of dopamine in this area is responsible for creating the feeling of immense pleasure and well-being. If you took one of your fingers and put it on the center of your forehead and another finger in the middle of the side of your head and drew a straight line from the end of each finger, where the two lines crossed would be the where the mesolimbic system is located in your brain. This area is also appropriately called our "reward center," and is essentially located deep in the center of our brains. It produces and stores the neurotransmitter dopamine. When dopamine is release and attaches to its receptor, we feel immense pleasure. This pleasurable feeling is interpreted as a reward, and this encourages us to repeat whatever behavior or experience is responsible for generating that feeling. Anything that ensures our survival as a species, such as sexual intercourse, finding and eating food, or having shelter and love, produces this reward and the feeling of pleasure, so we are encouraged to obtain it and/or engage in that activity. Anything that causes a release of dopamine in the mesolimbic system creates the sensation of pleasure, and the more dopamine released, the more pleasure one feels. Unfortunately, opioids, when abused or misused, are drugs that can cause a release of dopamine from the reward center in quantities that cannot be matched by any other real-life experience. The amount of pleasure experienced by the user can be perceived as greater than anything he or she has ever experienced. Because of this, using the drug can become habitual and lead to a chemical dependency and addiction. In fact, all chemicals and behaviors that are habit-forming and create a dependency or addiction, such as cocaine, alcohol, cigarettes, eating disorders, or sexual compulsion, do so by manipulating the release of dopamine in the reward center.

The opioids can do more than relieve pain and create a sense of well-being. They can also provide energy to the user, and relieve fatigue and depression. Early in my career of treating addictions, I would oftentimes have my patients tell me how Percocet gave them lots of energy. In fact, the laborers at construction sites nicknamed the drug "workacet." I related this to my own experience with Percocet, which I had been prescribed for severe pain, and how it had ultimately always put me to sleep. I was perplexed as to how these patients were getting energized from it, and was beginning to think there were people who responded differently to Percocet. Instead of getting tired and causing sleepiness, some people had the opposite reaction. It wasn't until I was suffering from a severe bout of lower back pain that I discovered something rather strange. Amid my excruciating pain and intense suffering, I took more pills than were prescribed, in an effort to relieve my unbearable pain. Much to my surprise, I reached a point where I felt an immense sense of calm and well-being. I had all the energy in the world, and my pain was completely gone. I realized I hadn't felt that good nor had so much energy in a very long time. I went about doing a lot of things that needed to be done that I had been putting off for quite some time. The funny thing was, my time spent doing the boring task, which I had dreaded doing, was actually very enjoyable.

It wasn't until later when this energized sense of well-being wore off that I realized this experience was the "high" my patients had been reporting. It wasn't some spaced-out, unable-to-function high that made one appear abnormal and unable to function; it was just the opposite. This feeling was very pleasurable and enabled me to get a lot of necessary work done. I was knowledgeable enough to know what was happening and to not repeat my actions, but someone who doesn't understand that he or she was getting high from Percocet may not know or want to stop. This person would continue to misuse the medication in order to feel energized, enhance performance at work and/or home, and feel better or relieve depression. What the patient wouldn't realize is that using the medication for this desired effect on a regular basis would only increase the likelihood that he or she would develop a dependency or addiction.

CHAPTER 4

WHY DO PEOPLE MISUSE OPIOIDS AND DEVELOP ADDICTIONS?

There are well-known mood disorders that people have which could make them susceptible to developing an opioid addiction. The medical literature tells us that 50 percent of the people who have addictions to opioids also have an underlying psychiatric illness (Watkins, 2004). In my experience, this could include but is not limited to, depression, anxiety disorders, bipolar disorder obsessive-compulsive disorder, attention-deficit disorder, personality disorders, and schizophrenia. The medical community has acknowledged that taking opioids while having underlying problems with anxiety and depression can make people prone to becoming addicted to them. There are also people with undiagnosed mood disorders who, out of ignorance and/or fear, have not sought medical treatment. Others might have stopped taking their prescribed medication because of undesirable side effects and/or lack of insurance or financial resources. Taking an illicit opioid can be a means of self-medicating and chemically coping with an undiagnosed and/or untreated condition. That's because opioids have a calming and soothing effect that can relieve depression, anxiety, difficulty sleeping, and posttraumatic stress.

Opioids can be abused and misused by adolescents, teenagers, and young adults in an attempt to relieve their social anxieties. It's very challenging growing up with all the peer pressure and competition our youth are subjected to. With the pressure to be socially acceptable, make friends, and be popular, it isn't hard to understand how some children can become stressed and feel anxious in certain situations. In social and intimate encounters, they may feel very awkward and unable to perform adequately. To relax, feel capable, and gain the acceptance of their peers, they might start experimenting with drugs. In the process they discover that they feel empowered by the opioids, which allow them to be calm and confident. With this type of positive reinforcement, opioid abuse can expand and become a way of chemically coping with the everyday stressors of life. It can become a habitual way of relieving boredom, loneliness, and a necessary ingredient for reward/pleasure-seeking activities. What starts out as a means of rapidly enhancing and improving one's mood can easily and unknowingly deteriorate into an opioid addiction.

People who have suffered a significant loss or traumatic event in their lives are prone to an opioid addiction. The unexplained loss of a loved one, loss of a job, financial ruin, and divorce can cause overwhelming emotional pain and suffering. Those subjected to physical and emotional abuse, rape victims, sexually abused children, and war veterans oftentimes battle anxiety disorders, post-traumatic stress and depression, and have anger issues. People don't always distinguish between physical and emotional pain, but these can both hurt and cause suffering. Opioid abuse becomes a way of numbing oneself and temporarily escaping the constant pain and fear. With habitual use, one can develop a psychological reliance, which over time can lead to a physical addiction.

Children raised by a parent who has an active addiction can grow up in a very chaotic and dysfunctional setting. Being constantly exposed to drugs and drug paraphernalia and witnessing firsthand the use of drugs, they become numb to the shock value. Activities involving drug use, and the resulting dysfunctional behaviors, become the norm and in some instances, a child's exposure to drug use is not by choice. One of my patients told me that her first encounter with heroin was when her uncle injected her with the drug when she was nine years old, and neither one of us could figure out exactly why he did it.

I have treated numerous patients with opioid addictions who were introduced to opioids by a physician, after an automobile, a slip-and-fall, or work-related accident or injury. They ended up being treated by a physician, receiving physical therapy, and filing a civil lawsuit against the party responsible for their injury. They had significant injuries, which caused debilitating pain, and were prescribed opioids to help relieve their ongoing pain and improve their ability to function in their everyday activities, improve sleep, and decrease their suffering. Oftentimes their injuries did not heal, and their pain and inability to perform certain activities persisted. After they settled the lawsuit, they were left with ongoing pain and became physically dependent on the opioids. The specialist who had been treating them for six months to two years discharged them with instructions to resume care with their primary-care physician. Many primary-care physicians do not feel comfortable prescribing opioids and refuse to do so; consequently, these patients are left with unmanaged, ongoing pain and a physical dependence on opioids. They are unable to find a physician to treat them and have to rely on friends, family members, or a drug dealer for their medication. Buying prescription painkillers such as Percocet and OxyContin from a dealer is very expensive. To generate the amount of money needed to support their habit, users engage in all sorts of risky, destructive, and oftentimes criminal behavior. Illicit drug sales range from forty to fifty dollars for each 80 mg OxyContin and ten dollars for a 10 mg Percocet. Depending on the amount of painkillers needed, a typical user can spend anywhere from fifty dollars to more than three hundred a day. Users experiment with heroin because it costs only ten dollars a bag, can be inhaled, and is more potent than the prescription painkillers. They soon find themselves rapidly increasing their use of the drug, going from one to two ten-dollar bags a day to more than twenty or thirty ten-dollar bags a day.

Many of the physicians who prescribe narcotic painkillers do not stress the perils of their use and just how easily patients can develop dependency or addiction to them. Patients need to be educated on how seductive and appealing the high from opioids can be. I instruct my patients that if their pain is gone completely, they have lots of unexplained energy, and their mood is great, they are probably high from the medication. Unfortunately, this is exactly the feeling a lot of people are looking for, and they become reliant on this feeling in order to function and can unknowingly develop a dependency or addiction.

Some people who develop an opioid addiction could be suffering from a speculative condition described as the "reward deficiency syndrome" (Blum, 1996). What this means is they don't make enough dopamine in the mesolimbic system in their brain, similar to people with depression who do not produce enough serotonin and norepinephrine. When they do initially take an opioid, they discover that their depressed mood, fatigue, aches, and pains that they had come to expect as normal are miraculously relieved. For the first time in their lives, they feel good. As of yet the medical community does not recognize this as a disease and therefore has no way of accurately diagnosing it, but that doesn't necessarily mean people can't be plagued by this condition.

CHAPTER 5

OPIOID DEPENDENCY

Many people mistakenly believe that as soon as an opioid user has withdrawal, he or she has an addiction, but this is not necessarily true. When people take opioids on a daily basis, their brain can undergo a process known as a neuro-adaptation, which means the anatomy of their brain has changed. The first sign of this change is when the user notices that the amount of opioid needed to obtain the desired effect has increased. This is known as developing a drug tolerance. The next change that might occur with neuro-adaptation is the development of withdrawal, or what users call being "dope sick." Withdrawals are very painful and described by users as being essentially intolerable. Sufferers present with tearing eyes, a runny nose, nausea, vomiting, abdominal cramping, joint and muscle pain, restlessness, anxiety, an inability to sleep, a sensation of being unable to tolerate being in one's skin, and restless kicking legs. The last symptom is responsible for the saying "kicking the habit," which has been used to describe the experience encountered when a user stops taking opioids. With the appearance of drug tolerance and withdrawal, the opioid user has now developed what the medical community calls a physiological dependency or opioid dependency.

Any drug that is ingested stays in the body until the body processes it and removes or eliminates it. This process is referred to as the body metabolizing the drug. For the body to metabolize a drug, it must first modify or break down the drug into different particles, and this action results in the drug being either activated or deactivated. When metabolized by the body, opioids are eventually deactivated in the liver and eliminated by the kidneys. When the human body deactivates a drug, that drug can no longer exert an effect on the body, and the body recognizes it as no longer being present. Each drug has a specific amount of time before the body metabolizes it and makes it inactive. The immediate-release opioids (Percocet, Vicodin, heroin, oxycodone, and fentanyl) are metabolized in three to four hours; the extended-release (OxyContin ER, Opana ER, and MS Contin ER) in twelve hours; Suboxone and Subutex in twenty-four hours; and methadone in forty-eight to seventy-two hours. If the user has a physiological dependency after the opioid is metabolized, he or she will start experiencing withdrawal. The withdrawal can start out mild and somewhat tolerable, but as time goes on, the severity increases. The withdrawal from opioids eventually becomes unbearable until the user takes more opioids. Users who have experienced withdrawal are usually deathly afraid of it. They usually do whatever it takes to get more opioids to avoid withdrawal, but having only drug tolerance and withdrawal does not mean the user has an addiction.

CHAPTER 6

OPIOID ADDICTION

A significant number of my patients have been convinced by friends and family members that they have an addiction when they really don't. People who take opioids for even a short time can experience drug tolerance to them and withdrawal. Having a tolerance causes the user to feel that he or she needs more medication in order to get the same benefit from taking it, so he or she requests it. Withdrawal may cause the user to panic and become preoccupied with getting opioids, but wanting more medication than previously needed and becoming anxious about not having it does not mean the person has an addiction. With an addiction a person not only has physiological dependence with drug tolerance and withdrawals but also an inability to function normally in his or her life. Users with addictions have lost control over their lives and spend a significant amount of time craving opioids. They continue to use opioids despite the detrimental effects and the destruction it causes to their health, work performance, and life. Distress occurs on the part of the user about his or her continual use of the drug, and the person repeatedly fails at attempts to stop using it.

When a patient has an opioid addiction, he or she is no longer taking the opioid for its intended use. Opioids are prescribed by physicians to relieve pain, but they can also be misused to relieve depression, anxiety, loneliness, and anger, and to help with sleep, provide energy, and relieve fatigue. Patients sometimes use them as a way of chemically coping with these undiagnosed and/or untreated medical conditions. When this happens the user might experience an initial relief of symptoms and a sense of wellness, but with continual use, some users' brains undergo neuro-adaptation. In a person with an opioid addiction, the brain no longer makes its normal amount of dopamine. The brain does this because the opioids the user has ingested have essentially taken over that job. When the opioids are metabolized or eliminated, his or her dopamine level drops below normal and the user's mood will deflate. This is referred to as a drop in one's "hedonic tone," and with this phenomenon, the feeling of unpleasantness persists. The person's dysphoria is accompanied by mild to severe withdrawal, and both can only relieved by ingesting more opioids. Unfortunately, the user's brain produces and releases so little dopamine on its own that when the person does use an opioid, he or she experiences no real high compared to those obtained before the addiction and the brain's neuro-adaptation. With this addiction the user is caught in the cycle of using opioids just to maintain comfort and stay out of withdrawal. He or she is caught in the vicious cycle of feeling the relief from withdrawal, with little or no high, and the panic and physical mayhem of the withdrawal.

In summary, if you are prescribed opioids for pain management and are taking them as often as directed and taking them only for pain, you do not have an addiction. If you notice that you are experiencing withdrawal in between taking the medication and/or after you completely stop taking it, you have a physiological dependency, or opioid dependency. If you are upset about your opioid use, are finding it difficult to function properly in your work and personal life while using opioids, are overly preoccupied with craving and obtaining the opioids, and are unable to stop in spite of negative consequences and/or harm to your health, then you have an addiction. If you have the symptoms of an addiction, but have convinced yourself that you don't have a problem and believe you can fix things whenever you want, then you are demonstrating one of the hallmarks of the disease of addiction—denial.

Patients suffering from pain and not being adequately medicated can appear to have an addiction. They might exhibit the behaviors of a user who has an addiction and engage in such activities as drug seeking, doctor shopping, and obtaining opioids illicitly from a friend or a drug dealer, but they don't have an addiction. They behave in this way because their pain is either not being treated, or not being treated properly or adequately. This condition is referred to in the medical community as a pseudo-addiction, and when patients are treated properly, their addictive behaviors cease.

CHAPTER 7

IS OPIOID ADDICTION A DISEASE?

If you have never had an addiction or have successfully overcome one, it is oftentimes hard to accept the fact that an addiction is a disease. A disease is a condition of the human body that impairs the body's ability to function normally and is associated with specific symptoms and signs. Medical research has proven that the brain of a patient with an opioid addiction has undergone changes in its structural anatomy and chemistry (Kalivas, 2002). These neuro-adaptations are associated with addictive behaviors and withdrawal. With this adaptation and change in the brain, using opioids is no longer a choice for the person, and the ability to control one's use of opioids is lost. For those with an opioid addiction, the reward center in their brains no longer produces enough dopamine to support normal bodily function. When the user doesn't ingest opioids, their chronically low dopamine level drops even further. This triggers an area of the brain called the "locus coeruleus" to be overstimulated and to produce excess catecholamines—adrenaline-type neurotransmitters—which contribute to signs and symptoms of withdrawal. Yes, an opioid addiction meets the medical criteria for a disease.

The prefrontal cortex is an area of the brain that is responsible for reasoning, logic, and problem solving. It does not develop completely in humans until the late teens and in some cases the mid-twenties. It is called the "executive center" because it allows for good judgment when making decisions and choices. The area of our brain where our emotions are centered and originate from is called the deep limbic system. For those with an opioid addiction, the connections between the prefrontal cortex and the limbic system are broken, and the ability to think rationally is taken away. Without the executive center's input, one has no thoughts about what is right or wrong, or about benefit or harm; there are just behaviors and actions coming from pure impulse, habit, and emotion. If a person develops an opioid addiction before his or her executive center has fully developed, the executive center stops growing. This person will have a tendency to respond to any craving or desire without thinking about the consequences and will exhibit the risk-taking and adventure-seeking behaviors common in one's teens and early twenties. This may in fact explain why the majority of people who have an opioid addiction are between the ages of eighteen and thirty-two.

People who have an opioid addiction are also susceptible to "triggers," which have traditionally been described as the people, places, and things associated with users' habitual opioid use. These triggers originate from the parts of the brain called the hippocampus and the amygdala. It is believed that the stimulation and release of the neurotransmitter glutamate is responsible for their development. When a trigger appears, glutamate is released in the hippocampus and the amygdala and then compels and motivates them to use. In the medical community, triggers are also referred to as "cues." Examples of cues can include: when stress builds up, when a user sees his or her drug of choice, when one is around the area where he or she used to buy drugs, when one sees people he or she used to get high with, or when a user sees someone who appears to be high. All of these triggers or cues create an uncontrollable desire in the user to get his or her drug of choice and use it.

When you have an addiction to opioids, the framework and the structure of the brain have changed, and the levels of neurotransmitters and their interactions are no longer normal. Every thought we have, every emotion we experience, and every action we take is based on the interaction among these different neurotransmitters and their receptors in our brains. When this system malfunctions, the negative changes to one's thoughts, feelings, and behaviors are devastating, and it's extremely hard for people who haven't experienced it to understand it.

Can those with the disease of an opioid addiction be cured? Yes, addictions can go into remission, but opioid addicts need to be careful and realize that they will probably have what I call a "lifetime allergy" to opioids. They could have years of sobriety and a normal life, but if they ever use an opioid again, they will probably suffer a relapse, and their disease will return as if it had never stopped.

CHAPTER 8

TREATMENTS FOR OPIOID DEPENDENCY AND ADDICTION

The first step, and oftentimes the hardest, is to acknowledge you have a problem and to admit that you have lost control over your actions. You don't want to use drugs, you've made multiple attempts to stop, and you know it's jeopardizing your health and ruining your life, but you can't stop. You can't control this disease; it controls you. After you do this, the next step is to realize that the way you have chosen to live is no longer working. Then you will come to the realization that some significant changes need to be made in how you choose to live your life. It also helps to surrender to the notion that you need some help and can't do it alone, but the one thing that will determine your success is how driven you are to get better. You have to want to get better so badly that you are willing to commit to making what could be very hard and drastic changes in the way you think and live.

One of the most tragic aspects of this disease is how the pain and suffering that comes from it can ripple throughout a family and have an impact on the people who love and care for the person with the addiction. One of the hardest things to do as a parent or an intimate partner is not to become what we call an enabler.

In most instances the feeling is to protect and shelter the addicted individual until he or she gets help or gets better. Unfortunately, you can love someone to death, and by not allowing the person to suffer the consequences of his or her actions, he or she will never be motivated to change. It's very hard to stand back and watch someone you desperately love hit rock bottom, especially when there are no guarantees that he or she won't end up dead or the victim of some horrific and tragic event, but that is exactly what you have to do. Otherwise, you become an enabler, and allow him or her to continue the addictive behavior without any losses or motivation to change. In some instances, your addiction becomes caring for the person, and you become codependent on his or her addiction. Feelings of love, guilt, and shame can lead to a code-pendency in which you attempt to control the user's life, but you must realize that this behavior only reinforces the disease. It can also give the user what is called a secondary gain, or a benefit, like your attention, which reinforces his or her need to use. You can't pressure, threaten, or berate the addicted individual to change. In fact, it can become counterproductive for you to yell and harass the person about what he or she should be doing, about how awful the person has been acting, and about how disappointed you are with him or her. Think about it: Has any amount of yelling, threatening, or outside pressure motivated you to make a signifi-cant change in your life? The decision to change must come from within the individual, and the outside pressure may only delay the process.

So how do you get someone to change? Well, there are differ-ent phases a person goes through while making a change in his or her life. The first phase is called the *pre-contemplative phase* of change. This is when someone is not even thinking about making the change. The second is when the person is thinking about making the change, and this is called the *contemplative phase*. The next phase is the *preparation phase*, when he or she starts taking steps to be prepared for the change, and when he or she actually makes the change, this is called the *action phase*. After an addicted person makes the change, he or she proceeds to the *maintenance phase*.

The trick for addicted individuals who seem bent on ruining their lives is to get them from the *pre-contemplative phase*, where they aren't thinking about not using, to the *contemplative phase*, where they are at least considering it. The way to do this is by giving them information that will start them thinking about it. Talk to them in a calm and nonjudgmental tone about the health risks of doing drugs, such as AIDS, hepatitis, endocarditis (infected heart valves), chronic sinusitis, and a weakened immune system. Give the person pictures, and tell stories of how the drug life has ruined people's lives, made them victims of crime, and brought physical harm and abuse upon themselves. Converting someone from the *pre-contemplative* to the *contemplative phase* of change is not an easy task, and it requires a lot of patience on your part, but it is effective. The knowledge you give the addicted person will push him or her into the contemplative phase, during which he or she is thinking about not using drugs, and this is where recovery from this disease begins. If you are not enabling the addicted individual, he or she will eventually suffer enough loss and pain and will realize what the problem is and ask for help. At this point it is time to prepare a plan to get professional help and then take the necessary steps to get it. You are now in the preparation phase of change, and as soon as the addicted individual attempts to stop using, he or she is in the action phase.

Both the person with the addiction and the people caring for him or her will have to persevere through this process and not allow frustrations and setbacks to deter them from continuing to fight this disease. There will be periods when the disease appears to be under control and the user stops using, which is called being in remission. This is the maintenance phase of change, which can be very challenging. The user may suffer a relapse and use opioids again. A relapse is usually very disappointing to all parties involved, but they are to be expected and are part of a normal recovery. What is important is that progress, however small, is being made and that no one stops trying. Suffering a relapse is like being knocked down in a fight. You can either stay on the ground and give up or get back up and continue to fight. If you want it really badly, you won't quit, and you'll continue to fight the good fight. Your attitude will determine your fate.

I've often said that life is very challenging, especially when one is growing up. There is the need for intimacy and companionship. You want to be accepted, fit in, and have friends, but many factors come in to play which influence one's ability to succeed. The type of parenting you receive and the environment you live in have an immense impact on the shaping your life. The funny thing is that we try so hard to control, but have very little say over what happens to us. You can't choose your parents or the neighborhood where you grow up. In fact the only thing you really can control is how you choose to respond to the daily events, situations, and challenges that confront you. Problems will occur, but your attitude about them will greatly influence your ability to overcome them. If you choose to numb yourself and escape from your problems, they will never go away and will only get larger. If you see the problem as an opportunity to make a significant change in your life and/or gain a valuable learning experience, that will make you a stronger and more capable person; then you will get through it and emerge victorious.

You can't force someone to seek help or change his or her life. That decision has to be made on one's own. People who have an addiction oftentimes have to hit rock bottom before they are ready to change their lives and get help. They must get to the point where they have nothing more left to lose but life itself, and then they finally make the decision to get help. For others, losing something of significance or value, or the threat thereof, is enough to motivate them to change. They can foresee impending doom, which motivates them to act. No matter what creates the desire to overcome an addiction and to change your life, it must be done with fierce determination. When my patients tell me they can't come to my office on a certain day, I ask them this question, "If I had a bag filled with a million dollars waiting here for you, would you get here?" They always laugh or smile, but they get the point that if they are properly motivated they will succeed.

Seed #1: If you want something badly enough, you'll develop a mind-set that says, "I'll do whatever it takes to get it, and I won't quit until I succeed." The amount of drive and effort you use to put into finding and getting your drug of choice you now must use to change your life.

An important and effective way to stay motivated is to define your purpose for living. This is what gives your life meaning, and you can choose what that purpose will be. Many people are confused and are waiting to find their purpose in life, but I tell them to stop waiting. You have the power to determine what that purpose will be *now*. You can chose to dedicate your life to raising a child, helping people with addictions, finding a cure for a disease, or building a successful business. You can decide now, and you don't have to wait. You can also change your mind and/or expand upon your original idea. You could also have multiple purposes with varying degrees of importance. It's solely up to you. The important thing is to get started and to overcome your fear of making the wrong decision or of failing. This is why finding a guide or a mentor is important, because not everybody has the ability to fly solo, especially in the beginning. There are many good people out in the world who enjoy helping others and who are not looking for, or don't need, anything in return. If good people see someone who is genuinely trying really hard to improve his or her life, they will usually want to help that person succeed.

If you need help in identifying this quality in yourself, look at the core strengths of your personality. I've often asked people, "Who are you?" Most people start reciting their profession, their age, their sex, and what they own. I remind them that material possessions and one's profession do not describe who we are. The great Greek philosopher Aristotle said, "Know thyself." I encourage people to take the time to sit down and figure out what their positive and admirable personality traits are. I ask them, "What are your noticeable characteristics that make you appealing to others? Are you trusting and/or passionate? Do you care about other people, like to organize things, and like to help other people?" After they have identified their positive traits, we then think of a profession, an activity, or a service in which these attributes could be best utilized. Some people might have to go back to their childhood and rediscover themselves before their pain, anger, and suffering occurred. Many times we make decisions about who we are based on our inability to stand up for ourselves, such as when we are children. In order to stop the pain, suffering, and ridicule, we become a person who is not our true self. Those decisions and changes may have worked then by protecting us and helping us to survive, but at the cost of our true identity.

The person we may have become is not who we really are, and by continually trying to be something we truly aren't, an internal conflict develops which robs us of our joy, peace, and serenity. Once you discover and acknowledge who you truly are, you can work at being that person and learning to love and appreciate your true self. If you have adapted and become something other than your true self, or if you are living out someone else's dreams, there will always be a deep-seated internal struggle. The battleground for this struggle is within you, and this internal conflict will manifest itself as pain and suffering in your life, which could ultimately lead to an addiction. Think about what you would choose to do if you knew you couldn't fail. Find a mentor or life coach who can help you come up with a plan to achieve your goal and/or help point you in the right direction. Don't be discouraged by feeling that the task is too difficult or not worth the effort. Remember how you use to persevere and how persistent you were when you were looking for drugs? The determination you need to be successful is already there, and it's been developed, tried, and proven. The only difference is that this time you are using it for something good and of benefit to you, and not for evil and self-destructive activities.

Seed #2: The greatest discovery in life is finding one's purpose, and for most of us, finding that purpose is a journey. Don't be discouraged if you cannot immediately define your purpose in life. If you approach this journey with enthusiasm and determination, you will ultimately find the love, acceptance, and quality of life you have been longing for. This leads to another important ingredient for your success: confidence. Confidence allows you to believe that your goals are obtainable, and without it the likelihood of achieving them is not good. You can gain confidence by building on each small success you have. The best way to succeed is to prepare properly, and choosing the proper medical treatment based on your individual needs is a good way to get started.

The first step recommended by most addiction specialists is to enter a rehabilitation center, where you can detoxify off the opioids and be educated on opioid addictions and the recovery process. The actual physical detoxification off opioids takes five to seven days, and the psychological rehabilitation twenty-one to thirty days. Whenever a chemical dependency associated with dysfunctional and destructive behavior develops, the first step should involve tapering off the drug in a safe environment under medical supervision. By putting the patient in a controlled environment, you can deny him or her access to drugs and monitor for any side effects and possible complications. If any problems develop, the patient can be quickly and effectively treated, thereby ensuring a more favorable outcome. It takes thirty days to break habitual behaviors and another thirty days to start new ones; consequently, the rehabilitation and the correction of the patient's behaviors are also very important. By putting the patient in a rehabilitation facility, he or she is removed from a lot of daily stressors, triggers, and responsibilities. Have you ever noticed how when you go away and leave your daily routine, you can see things more clearly? This new environment gives the patient a chance to reflect on his or her condition and to see things from a different perspective while also being educated about the disease and taught effective strategies to prevent relapse. This allows for the time and the opportunity to set up a support system that can serve as an ongoing resource to help with future questions and guidance. Unfortunately, not everyone can take advantage of the rehabilitation component due to time involved, financial and family responsibilities, and insurance difficulties. After the detoxification and/or rehabilitation process is completed, it is recommended that the patient continue with some form of counseling and medical supervision to help with any lingering withdrawal problems and/or cravings, and assist in structuring a life of abstinence. Programs exist that do intensive outpatient therapy/counseling for five days a week and gradually taper to three times a week, once a week, every two weeks, and then monthly. The National Institute on Drug Abuse (NIDA) of The United States Department of Health and Human Services states that for treatment to be effective it should last for a minimum of three months. I have found in my practice that a weekly counseling session for the first three months of treatment is a minimal goal, with the knowledge that the more time spent in counseling the better the outcome.

Many patients find that after their initial rehab and/or detox, their withdrawal symptoms are still there, and they can't control their cravings for the opioids. Withdrawal should normally last for only three to four days. When they persist for more than two weeks, this is medically referred to as the "post-abstinence syndrome." This condition of ongoing withdrawal can last for up to six months. Fortunately, with the post-abstinence syndrome, not all withdrawal symptoms are usually present, but one or two do linger on. It has been my experience that anxiety, restlessness, insomnia, and poor cognitive function (intelligence and memory) are the most common lingering withdrawal symptoms, but they do get better with time. Some of the withdrawal symptoms can be treated with prescription medications that relieve anxiety, nausea, vomiting, muscle aches, and restlessness, but if the withdrawal and/or cravings become overwhelming, the patient might need a crutch during the recovery process. This is no different than when a person breaks a bone and needs assistance, such as crutches, until the injury heals and the person gets stronger. Thankfully, Suboxone and methadone can assist a patient during his or her recovery and be the difference between success and failure.

Another option, which most third-party insurance companies will not pay for, and can cost between $5,000 and $10,000, is a rapid detoxification. In this option the detoxification is done under general anesthesia. The patient is unconscious and intubated and receives mechanical ventilation through a respirator machine. This procedure can also be done under intravenous sedation, where the patient is sleeping, but arousal can occur, and the patient is able to breathe on his or her own. The patient is given naltrexone, an opioid-receptor antagonist, which attaches to the opioid receptor and blocks the effect of any opioids. The naltrexone removes any opioids from the receptor sites and causes a rapid and severe withdrawal. Because the patient is unconscious, he or she does not feel the withdrawal, and after the procedure, the patient continues with naltrexone for up to twelve months. The problem is that *these patients might still crave opioids,* which may explain why historically this treatment has a very high early dropout rate, and not many patients stay with the treatment until its completion (Wodak, 2008).

Naltrexone can also be used without having undergone a rapid detox. It can be taken in the oral form on a daily basis or injected monthly. The injectable form is better because it lasts for a month, and the user is therefore less likely to suddenly stop taking the medication and relapse. It is manufactured by the Alkermes pharmaceutical company under the trade name of Vivitrol. It's hard to get started on naltrexone, because unless the patient is undergoing rapid detoxification, he or she must be absolutely opioid-free for seven to fourteen days before starting the medication. If not, the patient experiences severe withdrawal that cannot be reversed or relieved. Once on the medication, if the patient takes opioids, the euphoria is blocked, but if he or she takes too much opioid, to try to get high, overdose and death is possible. Worrisome side effects of naltrexone are mood changes, hallucinations, and suicidal ideation. When one decides to taper off the naltrexone and stop taking it, his or her opioid receptors can become hypersensitive. This means that if the person uses opioids, he or she could overdose and die on a much-lower amount of opioid than was previously used.

Recently, a non-opioid procedure for outpatient opioid detoxification was developed. In the study non-opioid medications—clonidine, which relieves physical withdrawal; lorazepam, for anxiety relief; and trazadone, which is a sleep aid and anti-depressant—and either a stimulant or no stimulant were used to complete outpatient opioid detoxification for 223 heroin-dependent patients. Overall, 61 percent of the patients successfully completed the outpatient detoxification and were transitioned to naltrexone maintenance treatment (Ockert, 2011). This study also demonstrated that naltrexone treatment is best suited for highly motivated patients, who are employed full time, have good social support, and have either private insurance or are self-pay patients (Ockert, 2011).

It's a good idea to get a psychological evaluation early on in one's recovery because 50 percent of the people who develop an opioid addiction have a co-occurring mental health disease. If a patient has one and doesn't get it treated correctly, he or she will always be inclined to self-medicate for that condition with the opioids. A mental health disease can be a contributing factor leading to the development of the addiction. In most instances the addiction to opioids should be treated first to see if any symptoms resolve with its treatment, because having mood disorders such as depression and/or anxiety resulting from the opioid addiction is not uncommon. That's why some physicians feel it's better to stabilize the patient first by treating the addiction and then allow him or her to become functional. If after six months any symptoms remain, an evaluation can be completed, a diagnosis can be made, and the appropriate treatment can be started. If the patient had a history of a mood disorder or the symptoms of one prior to developing addiction, chances are that it was not caused by the addiction, and an evaluation and treatment after one month of stabilization would be indicated.

The patient also needs to see his or her primary-care physician to get a comprehensive history and physical examination to detect any health problems that may have developed and gone undetected during the addiction. Communicable and infectious diseases such as hepatitis C and HIV can be successfully treated and have good outcomes. Data from the Centers for Disease Control and Prevention reveal that if the patient is an intravenous drug abuser, he or she has an 80 percent chance of being hepatitis C positive. Also, when the patient is hepatitis C positive, it does not mean he or she has a chronic hepatitis C virus infection. The screening test determines if the person has antibodies for the hepatitis C virus in his or her blood. If a patient is positive and has the hepatitis C virus antibodies, there is a 15 to 25 percent chance that the immune system was able to clear the virus from the body; consequently, 75–85 percent of the people infected with the hepatitis C virus will develop a chronic hepatitis C virus infection. Of the chronically infected, 60–70 percent will go on to develop chronic liver disease, 5–20 percent will develop cirrhosis of the liver over a period of twenty to thirty years, and 1–5 percent will die from cirrhosis of the liver. If a patient tests positive for hepatitis C, the next test would be a blood test called a "viral load," which would determine if the patient has any viral particles in his or her blood, and possibly a liver biopsy. The decision for treatment is based on the test results, and not every patient requires treatment. When treatment is recommended, in some instances the patient has a 75 percent chance of getting rid of the virus (Shiffman, 2007). There are also medications being developed that are more potent, require less treatment time, and have fewer side effects. If a patient does have hepatitis C, he or she can only transmit it through blood, and transmission through sexual intercourse is rare. The patient who is hepatitis C positive should also be vaccinated for hepatitis A and/or B virus, if tests for these return a negative result.

If a patient has completed a rehab and/or detox and has withdrawal symptoms and/or cravings that cannot be controlled, a good alternative treatment would be the drug Suboxone. There are also patients who for numerous reasons, such an inability to take time off from work, caregiving responsibilities at their home, confidentially concerns, lack of medical insurance, or an inability to self-pay, might feel a detox or rehab program is not a realistic option. Under these circumstances Suboxone therapy is a good option. Suboxone is a medication specifically approved for the treatment of opioid addictions that can be prescribed at a doctor's office visit. Doctors who prescribe Suboxone undergo specialized training, so they can be licensed by the DEA to prescribe the medication. My patients often refer to it as "a miracle drug," because it not only stops the cravings and withdrawals but it also makes them feel normal again, like they did before they started using opioids. Suboxone works like any other opioid by binding to the opioid receptor site, which relieves and prevents withdrawal and cravings but without causing a high.

Naloxone—one of the ingredients in Suboxone—is a generic drug that functions as an opioid blocker. Normally, when taken, it binds to the opioid receptor site, pushes off any other opioids that might have been there, and prevents any opioids from attaching to the receptor site. Like naltrexone, it does not stop cravings or withdrawal, but when attached to the opioid receptor site, it acts as a blocking drug by preventing other opioids from attaching and having any effect on the body. This drug is the same one given to patients who have overdosed on opioids, because it pushes them off the opioid receptor sites and reverses their action, but in doing so, it causes immediate withdrawal. Suboxone is taken sublingually (by placing it under the tongue) where it dissolves and gets absorbed there. The amount of naloxone in the Suboxone pill is such a small amount that it is not absorbed under the tongue, but if it is abused by being injected into a vein, it will work and cause immediate withdrawals.

Common side effects from Suboxone treatment are nausea, headaches, slower heart rate, drowsiness, excessive perspiration, and difficulty sleeping. The symptoms are usually mild and go away after two weeks. Constipation, which is also a common side effect of all opioids, may require a stool softener and/or laxative. Nausea, vomiting, and numbness and tingling in the arms and legs could indicate an allergic reaction to the naloxone, which would require a prescription of Subutex instead. You should not drink alcohol while treating an opioid addiction because it may weaken your resolve and allow for a relapse. Never combine the Suboxone with alcohol and any benzodiazepines such as Xanax (alprazolam), Valium (diazepam), Ativan (lorazapam, Librium (chlordiazepoxide), Klonopin (clonazepam), Restoril (temazepam), Halcion (triazolam), and Serax (oxazepam) because it can cause you to stop breathing while sleeping, and be fatal. Make sure your prescribing physician knows all the medications you are taking so he or she can prevent a toxic and potentially fatal complication from happening. If you develop drowsiness, your dosage of Suboxone might need to be lowered. It's also a good idea to be on a stool softener and increase your fiber intake with your diet to prevent constipation. Another common side effect from taking opioids is a low sex drive. This complication requires a medical workup consisting of a blood test and an MRI of the brain to see if there were any preexisting problems or tumors. It's been my experience that the results from these tests indicate that male patients will either need testosterone replacement or a prescription for Viagra or Cialis. The Viagra and Cialis not only relieve male erectile dysfunction but can also improve the male and female sex drive.

When starting Suboxone, the patient should wait a minimum of twelve hours, and preferably twenty-four hours, after last taking an opioid, which means he or she will be in mild to moderate withdrawal. Suboxone is classified as a partial agonist, meaning that it binds very tightly to the opioid receptor site; consequently, if there are any opioids in the patient's system when he or she takes Suboxone, the opioids will be pushed off the receptor sites and replaced by the Suboxone. If this happens, the patient's body will go into immediate and irreversible withdrawal. Irreversible withdrawals cannot be alleviated by taking opioids or any other medication, and the Suboxone will stay attached to the opioid receptor site for the next twenty-four hours. This is why I tell my patients to wait twenty-four hours after they last used an opioid before they start Suboxone so they can make sure all opioids have been cleansed from their system. Of course, there is one exception: If the patient has been taking methadone, he or she must wait three to four days—with four being preferable—after his or her last dose of methadone before starting Suboxone. Methadone stays in the patient's system for three to four days, and if the patient takes a dose of Suboxone before the body has had a chance to metabolize the methadone, he or she patient will go into immediate and irreversible withdrawal. At this point, the only thing the patient can do is wait it out or, if need be, go to the emergency room for observation and treatment. Physicians there can try to treat whatever withdrawal symptoms are problematic because there are medications that can relieve the nausea, anxiety, insomnia, muscle cramps, and restless legs, but the patient should not expect them to relieve all the withdrawal symptoms completely. If intolerable withdrawal occurs, I strongly recommend waiting for twelve to twenty-four hours and then resuming the Suboxone treatments. Nothing will really relieve the withdrawal, and using an opioid is a waste because its effect will be blocked by Suboxone. Waiting and bearing with the situation are the only things that will make your suffering worthwhile and purposeful.

When you are ready to take Suboxone, after waiting preferably twenty-four hours, you should be in mild to moderate withdrawals. Suboxone comes in a pill and film form in 8 mg and 2 mg sizes. Most patients are instructed to start with 4 to 8 mg. It should be placed under the tongue and left there until it dissolves completely. If you swallow Suboxone or spit it out, it will not get into your system and is equivalent to not having taken the medication at all. The film is the new-and-improved version of Suboxone, which dissolves much faster than the pill form and is preferred by an overwhelming number of patients to whom I have prescribed this medication. I prefer it because there is less chance of misuse, and the film removes the possible trigger of taking a pill. After the Suboxone dissolves, you should wait forty-five minutes to an hour to see if your withdrawal symptoms improve. If you are still in withdrawal, continue to take 4 mg to 8 mg every one to two hours until you have taken a total of two 8 mg pills/film. Over the first twenty-four hours, limit the amount of Suboxone you take to 16 mg. If afterwards you are still experiencing withdrawals and/or cravings you might need more Suboxone and can increase your daily dose by up to 8 mg for each of the next two days.

It is essential to remember that four 8 mg Suboxone (32 mg) is the maximum amount you should take over a twenty-four-hour period. The manufacturer of Suboxone tells us that the maximum dose should not exceed two 8 mg pills, but physicians have discovered that some people might initially need up to three or four pills and can safely take that many to relieve withdrawals and/or cravings. If these are not relieved, the likelihood of a patient continuing with Suboxone treatment diminishes greatly; therefore it is very important to rapidly extinguish withdrawal during the acute phase of the patient's recovery. Since Suboxone stays in your system and lasts for twenty-four hours, you have the option of taking your total dose all at once when you get up in the morning or dividing the total into two doses for the day. Most people with an addiction are used to using their drug of choice multiple times during the day and have developed a routine or pattern for their usage. I find it beneficial for some patients to somewhat mimic that pattern with the twice-a-day dosing, which psychologically can help control their cravings and urges to use. If the patient has difficulty sleeping, I recommend taking the second dose of Suboxone no later than six to eight hours before bedtime.

Most of my patients feel great on Suboxone and report that they feel the same way they did before they started using drugs. Others may have mild withdrawals for one to two weeks, but eventually they have that same good feeling. The important thing I tell my patients is to remember to take just enough Suboxone to relieve their withdrawal and cravings and no more than that. The goal should be to keep the dosage as low as possible, and my patients often find that after one to two weeks of treatment, the dosage can be lowered even further. Any patient initially requiring four 8 mg Suboxone should be able to safely and comfortably taper to two or three 8 mg Suboxone in one to two weeks. Unfortunately, some patients complain of intolerable and ongoing withdrawal and stop taking the Suboxone. This usually means one of two things: They started taking the Suboxone too soon and went into irreversible withdrawal and panic, or they were taking such a large amount of opioids on a daily basis that the Suboxone is not strong enough to stop their withdrawal and/or cravings. It has been my experience that patients who fall into the latter category are usually taking more than 320 mg of opioids (OxyContin ER, Percocet or Vicodin) or greater than 80 mg of methadone, or they are injecting or inhaling more than six ten-dollar bags of heroin a day. Patients who fall into this last category might need to taper their usage to less than those amounts before they start on Suboxone, because it might not be strong enough to control their withdrawal and/or cravings.

For these patients and/or those whose Suboxone treatment has failed, methadone treatment is a good option. Occasionally, when you mention the word *methadone*, some people get all sorts of distorted ideas and visions of safety hazards and health risk, based on unsubstantiated fears and mistaken information. The truth is, methadone, when administered correctly, is a very safe and effective treatment for opioid addictions, and it is the most extensively studied and regulated drug in America. Its use in the treatment of opioid addictions can only be done at a methadone treatment program that is regulated and licensed by the local, state, and U.S. federal government. The U.S. Government Accountability Office (GAO) released a report in April 2009 titled "Methadone-associated Overdose Deaths: Factors Contributing to Increased Deaths and Efforts to Prevent Them" to address a recent increase in methadone-induced fatalities. The report demonstrated that methadone deaths occurred in private physicians' offices, where methadone was being prescribed for pain management. Physicians cannot legally prescribe methadone in their private practices for the treatment of an opioid addiction, but they can prescribe methadone for the treatment of pain. Many physicians in private practice do not know that the first two weeks of methadone treatment can be very dangerous—even fatal—for the patient if the methadone is given too rapidly at a high dosage. The overwhelming majority of methadone-related fatalities occurred during the first two weeks of starting methadone treatment, because it takes time for the liver to get used to eliminating methadone from the body, and ingested methadone stays in the body for three to four days (GAO, 2009). That means that the day after starting on methadone, half of the methadone ingested the day before is still in the patient's system (Pate, 2002). If the methadone dose is increased too quickly, the patient can become over-sedated, have an overdose, and stop breathing. The methadone maintenance facilities have strict federal and state guidelines on exactly how much methadone can be given initially and just how rapidly a patient's dose can be increased. Depending on the patient's initial evaluation, the starting dose of methadone can only be 40 mg or less. Then, over the next seven to ten days, the patient must be examined by the medical staff and evaluated, to see if he or she qualifies for an increase or needs his or her methadone dosage adjusted based on their findings. Each day, patients are evaluated by trained medical staff under the direction of a licensed physician, and can make any adjustments or interventions deemed necessary. The ultimate goal is to safely get the patient to a dose where he or she is not craving or having withdrawals and has a blocking effect (no high) if illicit opioids are used. The average dose for those using methadone in America is between 60 and 120 mg, (Dole, 1966), but some patients could require a much higher dose for treatment success, sometimes exceeding 200 mg (Pate, 2003). What we don't want are signs of over-sedation such as drowsiness, confusion, and slurred speech, which means the dosage is too high. The patient should always be alert, oriented, and able to function without impairment. Some jurisdictions might even restrict driving while maintained on methadone, but the medical literature has shown that a patient who has been stabilized on methadone can operate an automobile safely and effectively (Lene, 2003).

There are two main advantages of a methadone maintenance program when compared to Suboxone treatment in a private physician's office. One is that the amount of methadone you can safely give to stop a patient's cravings and withdrawal is much higher when compared to Suboxone. The other is that the methadone maintenance facility also provides a more structured environment. Patients come to the facility each day for their methadone and can be closely monitored and observed. Problems can be more readily identified and can be acted upon in a timely fashion. Patients are referred to other healthcare professionals, are followed to make sure they keep their appointments, and are required to attend their individual counseling and group-therapy sessions.

Methadone treatment also remains the gold standard for opiate-dependent pregnant females, but high-dose Subutex (buprenorphine) has been accepted as a reasonable alternative, because a recent study showed there were no major differences between methadone and Subutex in terms of perinatal outcome (Lejeune, 2006). The U.S. Department of Health and Human Resources, Center for Substance Abuse Treatment Protocol (TIP 40) stated that methadone has been shown to be safe and effective for both the pregnant women and neonates, and that breast-feeding while on Subutex was not contraindicated. In my practice if a pregnant female is opioid dependent, being prescribed narcotic painkillers, and taking them as directed without any misuse, I recommend she continue taking them as prescribed. If a female patient on Suboxone becomes pregnant, she is converted to Subutex. If a female patient has an opioid addiction and treatment is started during her pregnancy, I recommend methadone treatment.

Initially, for safety concerns, patients in methadone treatment have to come every day to the methadone treatment facility to be monitored and receive their methadone. This practice might interfere with the patient's working schedule or personal responsibilities, but when a patient has stabilized and demonstrated an ability to appropriately manage his or her recovery, he or she can apply for a "take-home." A take-home means that the patient is given one of the daily methadone doses to take home, so he or she can administer it to themself the next day. That way the patient doesn't have to come to the methadone facility for one day. The decision to grant a take-home is made by a committee made up of the medical director, program director, counselor, and nursing administrator. The committee reviews the patient's performance and determines if he or she has met the state's and federal government's criteria for a take-home. This means that as the patient heals and no longer poses a threat to him or herself or to the community at large, he or she has the opportunity to be rewarded by not having to come to the clinic every day. Historically, patients that achieve a take-home usually stay in methadone treatment longer and have a better outcome (Peles, 2011).

Common side effects from methadone treatment are weight gain, excessive perspiration, constipation, drowsiness, and decreased libido. The drowsiness usually requires lowering the dose of methadone. Constipation is usually relieved by eating more fruits and vegetables, drinking eight eight-ounce glasses of water daily, and by taking a stool softener and/or laxative. A decreased libido requires the same medical work-up when it occurs with Suboxone and is usually, in males, due to a low testosterone level. The exact cause of this is unknown, but when present it can be easily treated with a testosterone replacement gel that is applied daily to one's skin. Women who suffer this complication are usually prescribed Viagra or Cialis, as are the men who fail with testosterone replacement. The weight gain that occurs with methadone treatment often shows up in the abdominal area. The exact cause is not known and could be related to poor eating habits and low activity levels that are comparable with the general population in America (Okruhlica, 2008). Addictive behaviors can lead to poor health and weight loss, but after the addicted individual gets treatment, he or she eventually stabilizes. With this, the patient's behavior normalizes, and he or she adopts lifestyle changes and/or replaces the drug reward with a natural one—usually food—which leads to a consistent increase in weight (Okruhlica, 2008). One-third of the adult population in America is overweight, and another third is obese. That means that two-thirds of the population in America is overweight, so one would expect two-thirds of the treated methadone patients to become overweight and a third to be obese. There is a product patients can purchase on the Internet called Vitadone, a vitamin and herbal remedy that, according to my patient testimonials, is effective in relieving many side effects associated with methadone use, especially the excessive perspiration and constipation. The weight gain can be effectively treated by professional nutritional counseling and an increase in exercise.

An opioid addiction is a disease of the brain, which changes the anatomy of the brain and how it works. Removing all opioids from the body by detoxing does not always fix the brain and make it work the way it did before the addiction. This is why after a simple detoxification, certain patients will continue to crave opioids and eventually relapse. Also, just replacing the abused opioid of choice with less toxic opioids such as Suboxone and methadone, and then not using, and living what appears to be a normal life might not be enough either. The only way to repair the brain and put the disease in remission is by replacing addictive thinking and behaviors with healthy thoughts and behaviors. The best way to do this is with counseling from a professional therapist skilled in the art of treating opioid addictions, and the more counseling you get the higher the probability of success.

To help explain this, I use this analogy with my patients: If you break a bone in your arm or leg and have a cast on it for six to twelve weeks, what does the arm or leg look like when you take off the cast? When you compare it to the side that wasn't broken and didn't have a cast on it for weeks, it is visibly smaller and appears to have shrunk. This is caused by atrophying; atrophy occurs when you don't use a part of your body, and the muscles and tissues shrink. When this happens, the patient starts physical therapy to strengthen the shrunken and weakened muscles, which makes them strong and healthy again. In a brain that has sustained an opioid addiction, the connections between the prefrontal cortex and the limbic system are not working properly and have essentially shrunk. The prefrontal cortex, under normal conditions, would tell us that even though opioid abuse might bring us immediate pleasure, it's a bad choice and not worth the risk. The prefrontal cortex would reason it's not a good decision to abuse opioids, and we would have the control not to do it instead of acting on impulse and emotion, and not weighing the consequences. The best way to repair and strengthen this area of the brain and to get it to function correctly is to participate in counseling, which is like doing mental push-ups or physical therapy on a weakened muscle.

I have found in my medical practice that for the majority of patients who seek professional help for an opioid addiction, the ultimate goals are to no longer have the need to rely on opioids in order to function, to be able to meet their responsibilities to themselves and their families, and to have a normal life. I tell patients that in order to accomplish these goals, they will have to rehabilitate their diseased brain back to a healthy neuro-anatomy and that the way to do this is to significantly change their thinking and behaviors. The change involves no longer believing that it's all right to rely on drugs to change their mood, manage stress, relieve boredom, comfort loneliness, and find a reward or celebrate. Going back to the image of the brain as an electrical circuit panel or motherboard of a computer, every thought and behavior you have has a chemical wiring laid down in your brain that must be used in order for that thought or behavior to happen. When someone has an opioid addiction that wiring is faulty, and he or she is essentially operating from a faulty circuit panel or corrupted motherboard. To fix the brain, we need to create a new motherboard or circuit panel from which the person can function—one that is constructed from healthy thoughts, moods, and behaviors, and one that can manage the daily challenges in our lives, reduce stress, relieve boredom, prevent feelings of loneliness and anger, and find a reward/celebration. Instead of operating from the old, diseased brain, we are creating a new, healthy one to work from.

CHAPTER 9

SEEDS FOR SUCCESS

At this point you should have a good understanding of what opioids are and of the nature of an opioid addiction. This is the solid foundation—a healthy soil laid down—so we can plant some more seeds that will enable us to do one of the most difficult and important tasks in one's life: change behavior. It's been my experience that many users with an opioid addiction believe two things very strongly: Their use of opioids is not a disease, and they could stop using if they were stronger and had more willpower. When they realize they can't do it, they feel guilty and have extremely low self-esteem and oftentimes end up disliking themselves.

Seed #3: You must understand that opioid addiction is a disease, that there is nothing to be ashamed of, and that it's important to stop self-loathing. We are not sure why some people can take opioids and not develop an addiction while others do. One thing is certain: When a user is caught in the throngs of his or her addiction, the person will clearly show that it is not a choice but a disease that happens to be like many of the other diseases that plague society. Labeling the people who have the disease by calling them "drug addicts" makes them feel guilty and ashamed. I believe that no patient should be referred to as a drug addict, because adding more shame and guilt by labeling that person an addict might not motivate the user to change and can only contribute to an acceptance of his or her condition as hopeless. Users with this addiction do challenge people with addictive behaviors that are quite obnoxious, offensive, and irritating, but we should understand these addictive behaviors are part of the disease process. Persons with an opioid addiction have little control over themselves and have faulty thinking and decision-making until treatment is started. Since a user who has this addiction oftentimes denies that he or she has a problem, and therefore does not seek help, the acceptance that he or she has an addiction is important, but calling the person a drug addict, or labeling oneself as such, can be counterproductive. It can contribute to the person's self-loathing, depression, and anxiety, which can cause a delay in the person's seeking treatment and/or prolong his or her recovery. People who have an opioid addiction need to take responsibility for their actions and not see themselves as a victim, which only makes their suffering worse. A bad choice may have been made, or they may not have been properly informed of, or understood the consequences of, their choices, but that alone does mean there is a flaw in their character. Good and honorable people make bad choices every day; it's just part of being human. Mistakes will happen, but the important thing is to first recognize that it happened and then try to understand how it happened so that corrective action can be taken to fix the problem and ensure it doesn't happen again.

Seed #4: You must believe that you can be successful in your recovery and accomplish all of your goals. Our beliefs are very powerful, and they will control the thoughts we carry in our minds throughout the day. The thoughts we have determine our mood, and our mood dictates our behavior. If you don't believe in yourself and doubt you will be successful, then you will have negative thoughts that will lead to a bad mood and poor behavior. If you do believe in yourself, your thoughts will be good and positive, and lead to a pleasant and positive mood that will manifest itself as good and productive behavior. You need to know and believe that either through you or through a power greater than you, your success is inevitable. It is just a matter of time, and all you have to do is *be patient.* The need for immediate gratification is part of human nature, but it is what might also have led to the addiction. With experience, you learn that taking shortcuts and trying to do things the fastest way possible can, in the end, create more problems than they solve. Good things and good outcomes require hard work and take time, and above all, you have to believe.

Seed #5: You must invest your whole mind, body, and soul into your recovery and be determined to succeed. When you decide to stop using, be passionate about it, but realize that not everyone will share this passion for your recovery. The harder you work at something and the more effort you put into it, the more you'll get out of it, but know that not everyone will want to hear about it or talk about it. Some people feel uncomfortable talking about drugs and don't understand why people use them, yet those same people might be in denial about their own abuse of substances such as caffeine, sugar, cigarettes, and alcohol. It's much easier for them to point their finger at you and find fault with you than address their own shortcomings. Other people are overwhelmed with their own struggles and challenges and don't necessarily want to hear about any more problems. So don't be surprised when other people do not want to share in hearing about your recovery, but don't let that rob you of your enthusiasm or diminish your efforts.

Seed #6: Start telling the truth all the time, and make a commitment to yourself to be an honest and trustworthy person. One of your most valuable assets is your personal integrity, which is the ability to have your speech and actions match your ideas and values. It means that you will not allow yourself to be corrupted and that you will walk it the way you talk it. When you live up to your decision to tell the truth and to be honest, you begin to regain your personal integrity. As you continue to gain strength and momentum, you start feeling good about yourself and realize that you never want to lose your personal integrity ever again, because what's more important than other peoples' opinions of you is how you feel about yourself.

Seed #7: Eliminate the triggers, people, places, and things associated with your opioid use. In some instances this is a very complicated undertaking, and for some users it can be very challenging. A user might not have the financial resources to move from his or her neighborhood, the opportunity to change jobs, or the ability or desire to sever a relationship with a loved one or financial provider. Some hard and painful decisions might need to be made, and the more successful you are at eliminating the people, places, and things that were involved with your addiction, the higher the probability you will succeed. Start by changing your cell phone number, and don't contact old acquaintances who were involved with your opioid use. As a replacement, develop a network of healthy friends, mentors, and family members you can rely on for support, love, guidance, and companionship. It's best to have different people you can go to for help, depending on your particular need or situation. Don't go to or even drive by places you frequented when you were using. Don't think you can be around drugs or people who are actively using opioids. Choose your friends and partners with great care. Understand your true value, and know what your needs are from a friendship or intimate relationship. Make sure the person who is receiving the gift of your friendship or intimacy is worthy of it, will appreciate it, and above all, is capable of fulfilling your needs.

Seed #8: Stop seeking pleasure, and start finding joy in your life. People want to be happy, but they must understand the difference between pleasure and joy, both of which can make us happy. Pleasure is short-lived, and after the feeling is gone, you will desire more. The problem is that when you are led by your desires and pleasure-seeking, you will never be truly satisfied. Joy is a feeling of calm and a state of serenity. It is a lasting happiness that prevails even amid ongoing difficulties and challenges. When I ask my patients which feeling they would rather have, they all choose joy. The best way to find joy in your life is by serving other people. I'm sure you have had the experience of participating in an act of kindness or of helping someone else. It makes you feel good and brings a sense of satisfaction and contentment, and you feel like you have accomplished something positive and worthwhile. It brings you joy. I encourage people to use this mind-set as they conduct their tasks during the day. When you are interacting with other people, don't concern yourself with how much recognition or reward you are receiving. Let your goal be to connect with people in a meaningful and helpful way. Encourage people, compliment them, and acknowledge the good they have done. If you can't find anything positive and good to say about them, then you probably need to avoid them, because instead of you lifting them up, they will probably just bring you down.

Seed #9: Find new and healthy activities to replace the activity of getting high using opioids. Getting a high from opioid abuse rewards the user with an intensely pleasurable feeling by causing the brain to release dopamine from the reward center, the mesolimbic system. Human beings have a basic need to reward themselves and to celebrate; however, when they become preoccupied and obsessed with relying on chemicals for this basic need, problems arise. Opioid abusers need to discover healthy activities that bring will them joy and a sense of accomplishment. Examples would be starting an exercise program, finding a hobby, reading, and engaging in an educational program. The more knowledge-able individual will be better equipped to develop effective coping skills and a sense of satisfaction with their lives. Also, make sure there is a healthy balance between work, family responsibilities and commitments, and recreational activities. Many people get caught up in doing things for others and neglect themselves, and as time progresses, they lose their sense of self and start feeling overwhelmed and unhappy. Get a daily planner and schedule time for yourself when you can take care of your own personal needs and bring a sense of joy and personal satisfaction to yourself. It's not being selfish, but by learning how to say "no," you won't be overwhelmed with other people's needs and problems. You will be less stressed, have more energy and enthusiasm, and will be more productive when you do take care of your daily responsibilities.

Seed #10: Make a decision to stop taking risks and going to extremes. As you look back on your life and analyze it carefully, you might discover that you take risks and like thrills or extremes. Initially, a risky adventure might bring a thrill and give the illusion of being worthwhile, but if you examine it carefully, you will see that this type of behavior ultimately ends up causing you to suffer. If you want to stop suffering, then stop taking risks that could jeop-ardize your health, lead to legal problems, or cause significant per-sonal and/or financial losses. Understand that more is not always better and that going to the extreme more often than not creates a toxic situation that leads to more suffering. Realize that if you continue to take risks, you will just be on an endless quest filled with chaos, turmoil, and possible catastrophic loss.

Seed #11: Learn to turn a negative into a positive by refram-ing your painful experiences. One thing an opioid addiction will eventually do is bring you down to your knees and make you realize that life can throw you some real surprises. It is a very humbling experience, but the upside of this is that by being humbled you are less apt to judge others and you become more tolerant of other people's mistakes. Life starts to slow down and you develop an appreciation for less without always craving more. Have you ever noticed how the right frame on a picture can make an average picture look great? In the same way, you can learn to reframe your failures as valuable learning experiences that are responsible for your ultimate success. Our successes in life usually teach us very little, but we can learn a lot from our failures. We learn to persevere and endure and develop the maturity and character needed to be successful at reaching the goals in our lives. When we do reach our destination, we appreciate it more and are less inclined to risk losing it.

Seed #12: Understand that wealth and good fortune are things you attract. Grow to the point where your thoughts, speech, and actions are honorable, pure, and consistent with one another. Keep your thoughts positive and pure, and don't speak crudely or engage in negative conversations or activities. Do the right thing as you interact in the world and treat people the same way you want to be treated. When you chase something, you usually end up exhausting yourself, and when you do get it, you realize that it wasn't what you expected. When your thoughts, speech, and deeds are all positive, you attract positive things back to you. Doors of opportunity no longer have to be kicked down, because they will open for you on their own, and you will realize that a door that needs to be kicked open is not the correct path for you. You don't have to take risk or force things; just be patient and wait for the right opportunity, which will reveal itself as a gift.

Seed #13: Stop wanting and start living. Take control of your thoughts in the morning when you wake, and set the tone for your day by dedicating yourself to one simple task. Instead of dwelling on what you want or worrying about what needs to be done, think of all the things you have to be grateful for. In your mind's eye, list them one by one. Perhaps you are thankful for your life, loved ones, food, shelter, and the many things you already have and take for granted. Be grateful, and acknowledge the blessings you already have. After that mental exercise, make a commitment to stop wanting things. Continue to make plans and do the things you need to do, but amid fulfilling your plan, stop thinking about wanting or doing something else. When you dwell on wanting something, you take yourself out of the moment and can't enjoy and appreciate what's right in front of you. You spend your time rushing, feeling unfulfilled, and worrying about things in the past and/or future and miss out on experiencing the potential joy in the present moment.

Seed #14: Stop worrying. Worrying is fruitless because you are spending your precious time trying to get control of a situation you can't control, so you continue to replay all the scenarios and options in your head without solving the problem. Take a moment to think of all the problems you have encountered in your lifetime. Didn't they all eventually work themselves out? Did the worrying ever help solve the problem or make you feel any better? Have faith that after you have done all you can that things will eventually work themselves out, and that no matter what happens, you'll get through it and survive. If worrying or excessive thinking is interfering with your sleep, schedule about a half-hour during the day when you can think your problems through. Make sure all feasible options have been considered, and that you have tapped into all of your available resources. Exhaust all logical possibilities, develop a plan of action, and then stop thinking about it. Then when it's time to sleep and things have settled down, you won't start problem solving or worrying because you will have already done that.

Seed #15: Do not be self-reliant when it comes to your recovery. Being self-reliant is having the belief that you know what is right more so than anyone else that you don't need any help, and that you can do it better by yourself. Self-management is a big part of the recovery process, but that doesn't mean you don't need help from other sources. Help can come in the form of reading literature about the addiction, individual counseling, group therapy, and/or a life coach. If you are hesitant to reach out for assistance and you wonder if it will make a difference, I strongly recommend you at least try two to three of these sources of help for at least three months, and then judge for yourself.

The twelve-step program is a valuable undertaking and can become a significant part of a solid support system. Narcotics Anonymous, which was founded and is operated by opioid abusers who developed an addiction and are in recovery, is considered a self-help program. There are twelve steps that each participant is encouraged to work on, and when the steps are completed, the participant will have transformed from an opioid abuser into a new person. There are also support groups for the family members of recovering opioid users. Meetings are held multiple times during the week, at convenient hours and in a group setting. I encourage people who want to participate to initially visit one and see if it's for you. If it is then pick a sponsor and get to work on the twelve steps. Just going to a meeting to listen to what people have to say, and socializing, are not enough; you must work on the twelve steps. People who have anxiety in social settings might not feel comfortable in the group setting. I would encourage them and others who can't participate to purchase one of the many available books that explain the twelve steps and offer instructions about how to do them. Any questions and feedback can be done with an individual therapist or experienced mentor.

In the twelve-step program, participants are expected to abstain from drugs and using drugs such as methadone or Suboxone to aid in one's recovery may be frowned on. The first step is to admit you have a problem and have lost control over your life, and the second is to believe in a higher power and to submit to that power. As a born-again Christian and ordained minister, I can personally attest to the ability of using this belief to overcome any obstacle in one's life. Some twelve-step followers end up coming to Christ, while others put their faith in a higher power. You no longer have to rely on your own power to overcome the addiction, but have a higher power to assist you. Your thoughts and behavior adjust and change and you find yourself staying away from extreme behaviors motivated by pride, jealousy, selfishness, and anger.

One thing you don't want to do is substitute one chemical dependency for another. Caffeine is the number one chemical dependency in America. Drinking excessive amounts of coffee and caffeinated beverages can increase anxiety, make you irritable and easily fatigued, and interfere with sleep. Smoking tobacco can lead to a nicotine dependency. The U.S. Centers for Disease Control and Prevention reported statistics from 2000 through 2004, that tobacco is the leading preventable cause of death and is responsible for about one in five deaths annually. This amounts to approximately 443,000 deaths per year, and an estimated 49,000 of these tobacco-related deaths are a result of secondhand smoke exposure. On average, smokers die thirteen to fourteen years earlier than non-smokers. The nicotine patch or prescription medication Chantix (varenicline), when combined with counseling, has a high success rate for smoking cessation. I always recommend the nicotine patch first because of the reports of nightmares, aggressive behavior, and suicidal ideation as potential side effects from using Chantix. Be careful not to find a reward in eating junk food, which is usually high in carbohydrates/sugar and saturated fats, or in overeating, which can lead to obesity. Heart disease is the leading cause of death in America, and the high cholesterol, high blood pressure, diabetes, and a sedentary lifestyle that can accompany being obese are a major cause of heart disease. If you have any of these issues in addition to an opioid addiction, consider treating them all simultaneously. People who treat all of their addictions and dependencies simultaneously change their core beliefs about their need for all unhealthy substances and poor habits, and by eliminating them all at once, they are making a more thorough and stronger commitment to change, which should lead to a better outcome.

The length of time you need to stay on Suboxone or methadone depends on individual circumstances. What's important is that changes have been made in how you think, how you feel, and how you act. Your character will undergo a significant change for the better, and knowledgeable people who truly know and care for you will notice this and compliment you on your changes. Instead of being obsessed with using opioids and devoting a majority of your time either using or obtaining opioids, you will have found a healthy and beneficial activity to replace your opioid use. You will have made a sincere effort and accomplished to the best of your ability eliminating the people, places, and things from your life that were associated with your use of illicit drugs. You will have developed healthy behaviors and learned techniques for managing stress, relieving boredom and loneliness, soothing and preventing anger, and celebrating or finding a reward in lieu of relying on chemicals or drugs. Stress will always be there in varying degrees, and you will have good days and bad days. Eventually, no matter how appealing and fulfilling the new routine is, boredom will creep in. You are going to need a release and seek a reward and/or celebrate. You will need a well-balanced life with legitimate and healthy ways of having fun and breaking the monotony. You will then have accomplished the desired changes and will have your new life. You must then live it successfully for a minimum of sixty days, and the longer, the better. By changing how you think, feel, and behave, you will have created that new circuit panel or motherboard in your brain and will now be operating from it. The disease, with its cravings, will be in remission, so you can be tapered off the Suboxone or methadone and expect only physical withdrawal, which will be less severe than those complicated by emotional withdrawal. The only thing left to do will be to make sure you have a good support network in place and use it.

CHAPTER 10

MANAGING WITHDRAWAL

Attending a facility for a five-to-seven-day chemical detoxification is an acceptable way to launch this part of your recovery. When you finish your detox and are released, you will still have challenges, but you will have overcome a major hurdle. You can build on the momentum generated from accomplishing the goal of being off all opioids, and successfully continue with your journey. If you are taking Suboxone, I recommend being on a dose of 2 to 8 mg; if you are taking methadone, it should be a dose of 20 to 30 mg for at least thirty days with the lower doses preferable.

Detoxing off Suboxone or methadone can also be done safely and successfully as an outpatient. The methadone withdrawal is reported to be more severe and usually requires more time. I recommend lowering one's methadone dose by 1 to 5 mg every ten to fourteen days. When withdrawal and/or cravings become intolerable, then stop the taper, and wait fourteen to twenty-eight days before you attempt to resume your taper. When you reach 80 to 30 mg of methadone, you have the option of transferring to Suboxone. Most physicians prefer you be at 30 mg, but a medical study involving over one hundred sociologically and socially stable patients receiving methadone maintenance treatment determined that transitioning from methadone on doses up to 80 mg to Sub-oxone is generally well tolerated, and that Suboxone is efficacious, safe, and well tolerated long-term (Salsitz, 2010). The most important and difficult part is that you must stop taking methadone for three to four days before starting Suboxone. If you start too early, you will have severe withdrawal that cannot be relieved by taking an opioid or any other drug. If this happens, just continue to take 4 to 8 mg of Suboxone every twelve hours for twenty-four hours. After twenty-four hours, the worst will be over, and you can advance your dose as need to relieve any lingering withdrawals or cravings. Transitioning from methadone maintenance treatment to Suboxone treatment usually allows the methadone patient, who might have had a more extensive drug history, greater freedom and more responsibility without suddenly introducing him or her into a new environment without adequate professional support and monitoring.

With the Suboxone detoxification, the taper can be done by lowering the dose by 1 to 4 mg every fourteen to twenty-eight days. Once again, when and if withdrawal and/or cravings become intolerable stop the taper until the symptoms resolve. Be patient, and do not try to force the issue. Your body makes its own opioids through your endorphin system. When you are supplying opioids from an outside source, your body doesn't need to make its own endorphins, and the system can shut down and go to sleep. As you lower your dose of Suboxone or methadone, your endorphin system has to wake up and start working again. This is a process, and it can take time. Shocking or jump-starting your system with a rapid decrease in the amount of Suboxone or methadone usually doesn't work, because the withdrawal from doing so proves to be too harsh and intolerable. Your withdrawal might also have an emotional or psychological component, which can force you to stop your taper so you can do more internal work on yourself and make the necessary behavioral changes before you can resume your taper. It's important to be patient, acknowledge your improvement at a lower dose, and realize that you are getting closer to your goal.

Patients who at one time had chronic pain issues might discover that their pain that was once removed with higher doses of Suboxone, and especially methadone, is now returning. Chronic pain is characterized as pain that lasts for greater than three months, and some patients who have chronic pain have tried the best of what traditional medicine has to offer and have only found relief from their pain with prescription medication. I have treated countless patients with chronic pain and have endured ongoing pain myself due to multiple herniated discs with damaged nerves in my neck. Many times nothing in modern medicine can cure the disease; when this happens, you have to heal yourself. You start by controlling what you can by engaging in beneficial lifestyle changes and learning to control your thoughts. If you smoke cigarettes, you have to stop. Your body cannot heal itself if you are constantly dumping all sorts of toxins and poisons into it. Smoking cigarettes also destroys the circulation to your body's tissues, and the oxygen and nutrients these tissues so desperately need in order to heal can't get there. Smoking cigarettes essentially accelerates the disease and makes it worse. You need to have a good level of overall physical conditioning, which usually means, for most people, improving flexibility, muscular strength, stamina, and cardiovascular conditioning (aerobic exercises). Your nutritional needs must consist of a well-balanced diet of healthy food, with proper portions, at correct times, and lots of water.

There are also home remedies (alternating ice and heat treatments, tiger balm and bio-freeze), physical therapy treatments (ultrasound, electrical stimulation, myofascial release and thera-peutic injections), medical equipment (tens unit, specialty bed and whirlpool), and alternative medical treatments (rolfing, yoga, tai chi, palates, and acupuncture) that can improve your condition and quality of life. Keep an open mind, and try different options. You must also learn to not allow your pain to gain all of your atten-tion and to find enjoyable and engaging activities to consume your time. If you have done all of this and still have some pain that interferes with your ability to function and/or to sleep, and severely affects your quality of life, then you might need to stay on Suboxone or methadone at the lowest dosage that relieves your pain to a moderate level and allows you to function on a daily basis without suffering.

Some patients might also want to try the inpatient rapid detox-ification under anesthesia, or the outpatient non-opioid detoxi-fication using clonidine, trazodone, lorazepam, with or without a stimulant (Ockert, 2011). Whether or not the patient who has already undergone extensive counseling and has been abstinent from illicit opioids for over six months would require naltrexone therapy afterwards can be determined on an individual basis by a team of medical and counseling professionals.

Withdrawal from opioids normally lasts from three to seven days, but it can also be protracted and last from six weeks to six months. The condition of protracted withdrawal symptoms is the post-abstinence syndrome. Continuing with counseling and hav-ing a good support system and qualified medical intervention can help with this problem so that you can maintain healthy behaviors and have constructive and positive thoughts during this process. There are prescription medications and herbal remedies that can help with the symptoms of withdrawal. Clonidine is a prescription medication originally used to control high blood pressure and has been found to be effective in relieving withdrawal. A study published in the Journal of Clinical Pharmacy and Therapeutics in 2001 reported that the combination of clonidine and the herbal remedy passion flower had beneficial results. The clonidine alleviated the physical withdrawal, and the passionflower alleviated the mental symptoms such as anxiety, agitation, and irritability (Clark, 2010). The herbal remedy *Nigella Sativa*, known as black cumin or fennel flower, at dose of 500 mg three times a day has also been shown not only to relieve withdrawal and cravings but to help improve any associated weaknesses and infections (Sangi, 2008).

Other prescription medications exist that can help with symptoms such as nausea, vomiting, restless legs, abdominal cramping, and muscle aches. A qualified and experienced physician, after listening to the patient and determining which withdrawal symptoms are problematic, can prescribe the appropriate medication at the correct dose and time of day. Anxiety, excessive nervousness, and insomnia are common problems that have historically been treated with a group of drugs called benzodiazepines, but the decision to prescribe or take benzodiazepines for longer than three or four months should be considered carefully. Benzodiazepines have been highly prescribed by physicians in America since the first benzodiazepine, Librium, was manufactured in the 1960s. The National Institute of Mental Health reports that benzodiazepines are generally prescribed for short periods of time, especially for people who have abused drugs or alcohol and who become dependent on medication easily (2009). Patients who have been taking benzodiazepines for longer than three or four months can develop a very dangerous physical dependency to them. Benzodiazepines' effectiveness at relieving anxiety and insomnia will decrease over time, and a patient with a dependency to them will experience a very uncomfortable withdrawal when they try to stop taking the medication. The withdrawal includes the original symptoms of anxiety, nervousness, and insomnia that the benzodiazepine was intended to treat, but it is magnified two to threefold. This is called a "rebound effect" and might discourage a patient from feeling that he or she can successfully stop taking the medication. An even bigger problem is that if a patient were to stop taking the benzodiazepines suddenly, he or she could have a life-threatening seizure. Benzodiazepines are also commonly abused by individuals with opioid addictions, because users can enhance the high they get from misusing opioids. The benzodiazepine Xanax—alprazolam, generically—comes in a bar that users and dealers call a "xanny bar." Because Xanax reaches the brain very rapidly after being ingested, it has a high abuse potential. It is commonly misused by opioid abusers to enhance the euphoria from their opioid misuse. Patients receiving methadone have reported that using benzodiazepines like Xanax before or immediately after receiving their methadone can mimic the high from heroin. Misusing benzodiazepines and opioids simultaneously can severely impair one's ability to function and/or can lead to a life-threatening overdose. The first line of prescription medication used in the treatment of patients with anxiety disorders is usually one of the newer antidepressants called selective serotonin reuptake inhibitors (SSRIs). Cognitive and behavioral therapy from a trained therapist can be even more effective in relieving anxiety and insomnia for some patients.

CHAPTER 11

CONCLUSION

An opioid addiction is a very complicated disease with multiple components. It is oftentimes associated with other potential problems, including chronic pain; a mood disorder such as depression, anxiety, bipolar, obsessive-compulsive, attention-deficit; a sleep disorder; a dysfunctional family setting; and side effects from prescribed medications. The best advice, amid what can appear to be an overwhelming situation, is to remember to simplify things. Initially, the major focus of one's recovery should be to stop using opioids and stay clean. This is called the acute phase, and **after thirty days of abstaining from opioid use, the disease (addiction) is in remission**. Above all, be patient with the speed of your recovery, and remember that relapses are part of the recovery process. Don't be your own worst enemy by being too harsh with yourself. Stay positive and build on your experiences, good and bad, by learning from them. Bad behavior is the result of poor choices, which is based on faulty thinking. With proper guidance you can learn how to think effectively so you can make good choices and develop healthy behaviors. As you progress, your focus will no longer just be on stopping use, but on learning to view yourself and the world around you more positively. You will be able to change your thoughts, speech, and behavior from bad and destructive to good and nurturing. You will resonate positive energy and attract wealth and prosperity. Start by doing what your chosen opioid addiction experts (trained counselors, qualified physicians, and experienced mentors) are telling you to do, without trying to add to or subtract from it. As you experience the benefits from the lessons learned, you will start to understand why your recovery has to be done a certain way. You will come to believe in what you are doing, and at that point, the changes you have made will become a part of you. When circumstances surrounding you become difficult and you are tested, the new and positive beliefs rooted in your spirit will enable you to overcome old obstacles and meet new challenges. Your dignity and personal integrity will prevail and carry you through any difficulty.

Seed #16: Don't just do the right thing; do it for the right reasons. The decision to change comes from a change in one's heart. During the process of contracting and then living with an opioid addiction, one's heart can become hardened and resistant to change. For some it's only after significant losses that they are humbled, their heart softens, and they allow themselves to accept and seek change. With a humble spirit and a pure heart, examine the motives behind your actions. Be honest with yourself, and make sure your intentions are rooted in advancing not only your own self-interest, but also in helping, and not hurting, others.

The most valuable thing you have is your time, and stop wasting it, because once the moment passes, it's gone forever. You can spend your whole day wanting to be somewhere or wanting something you feel you need. When you finally get what you want, you start wanting something else, and it becomes a vicious cycle of constantly wanting what you don't have. If what you want brings you pleasure, the wanting can turn into craving, and then the seed of an addiction has been planted. All that time spent wanting also keeps you from being in the moment and being aware of your surroundings. You are unable to enjoy the part of your life that is right in front of you, because you are somewhere else in the past or future wasting the precious moments of the here and now. Living in the moment allows you to appreciate its beauty and take advantage of its opportunities. If you had one day to live, what would you do that day? I suspect you would spend that time with your loved ones. The things that annoy you would evaporate, and to get the most out of your time left, your focus and attention would be in the moment. When you are in the moment, worry and doubt disappear and are replaced with calm and tranquility. When you stop doubting yourself, what you believe in will materialize. You can still have goals in your life and develop strategies on how to achieve them. When the time presents itself for you to carry out your plan, just do it.

With determination, hard work, and help from experienced and knowledgeable professionals, an opioid addiction can be overcome. Everyone gets another chance, as long as he or she gets up, dusts him or herself off, and doesn't quit. No one ever asked to get this disease, but you can choose to do something about it. The victory is yours to claim by just making the decision to change and by committing yourself to do the right thing. Discover the warrior spirit that's inside of you, and fight for your life, earn respect, attract good fortune, and, by all means, embrace the journey. Don't stay rooted in old habits and behaviors that clearly do not work anymore. Be aware of the choices you make, their consequences, and learn from your mistakes. Repair yourself by creating and managing a therapeutic recovery that will allow you to adapt to the challenges in life in a positive way. Do more than just survive, and instead evolve into a well-balanced, complete, and joyful person with a rewarding quality of life.

REFERENCES

Aggrawal, M.D., Anil. "Chapter 2: The Story of Opium. *Narcotic Drugs*. New Delhi, 1995. Print.

"Annual Smoking-Attributable Mortality, Years of Potential Life Lost, and Productivity Losses- United States, 1995–1999." *Centers for Disease Control and Prevention*. Morbidity and Mortality Weekly Report, 2002. Web.

Blum, Kenneth, John G. Cull, Eric R. Braverman, and David E. Comings. "Reward Deficiency Syndrome." *The American Scientist* (1996). Web.

Booth, Martin. *Opium: A History*. London: Simon & Schuster, 1996. Print.

Clark, Brian. "Passion Flower and Clonidine for Opiate Withdrawal." *Health & Wellness*. Associated Content, 22 Mar. 2010. Web. <www.associatedcontent.com>.

Claude, Lejeune, Laurence Simmat-Durand, Laurent Gourarier, and Sandrine Aubisson. "Prospective Multicenter Observational Study of 260 Infants Born to 259 Opiate-dependent Mothers on Methadone or High-dose Buprenorphine Substitution." *Drug and Alcohol Dependence* 82 (2006): 250–57. Web.

"DEA Imposes 'Emergency' Ban to Control Synthetic Marijuana." *CNN*. 28 Feb. 2011. Web.

"Driving Okay for Methadone Users." *About.com*. Elsevier Science News Release, 2003. Web.

Fishbain, D.A., H.L. Rosomoff, and R.S. Rosomoff. "Drug Abuse, Dependence, and Addiction in Chronic Pain Patients." *Clinical Pain* 8.2 (1992): 77–85. Web.

"Hepatitis C FAQs for the Public." *Centers for Disease Control and Prevention.* Web. <www.cdc.gov>.

"How China Got Rid of Opium." *Society for Anglo-Chinese Understanding.* Web. <www.sacu.org/opium>.

Kalivas, Peter W. "Neurocircuitry of Addiction." *Neuropsychopharmocology: The Fifth Generation of Progress.* 2002. 1357–363. Print.

Latimer, Dean, and Jeff Goldberg. *Flowers in the Blood: The Story of Opium.* New York: Franklin Watts, 1981. Print.

Marshall, Edward. "Uncle Sam is the Worst Drug Fiend in the World." *New York Times* 12 Mar. 1911. Print.

McCoy, Alfred. *The Politics of Heroin: CIA Complicity in the Global Drug Trade.* New York City: Lawrence Hill, 1991. Print.

Muller, H., and W. Sperling. "The Synthetic Cannabinoid Spice as a Trigger for Acute Exacerbation of Cannabis Induced Recurrent Psychotic Episodes." *Schizophrenia Research* 118 (2010): 309–10. Web.

Musto, David F. *The American Disease: Origins of Narcotic Control.* New York: Oxford UP, 1987. Print.

Ockert, David M., Joseph R. Volpicelli, Armin R. Baier, Jr., Edgar E. Coons, and Alexandra Fingesten. "A Nonopioid Procedure for Outpatient Opioid Detoxification." *Journal of Addiction Medicine* 5.2 (2011): 110–14. Print.

"Opium Throughout History." *Frontline PBS.* The Opium Kings. Web.

"Opium Throughout History." *The Opium Kings.* Frontline PBS. Web.

Payte, J.T. "A Brief History of Methadone in the Treatment of Opioid Dependence: A Personal Perspective." *Journal of Psychoactive Drugs* 23 (1991): 103–07. Web.

Payte, J.T., J.E. Zweben, and J. Martin. "Opioid Maintenance Treatment." *Principles of Addiction Medicine* (2003): 751–66. Print.

Payte, J.T. "Methadone Maintenance Treatment: The First Thirty Years." *Journal of Psychoactive Drugs* 29 (1997): 149–50. Print.

Payte, J.T. "Opioid Agonist Treatment of Addiction." *ASAM Review Course in Addiction Medicine.* 2002. Web.

Peles, Einat, Shaul Schreiber, Rachel Bar-Hamburger, and Miriam Adelson. "No Change of Sleep After 6 and 12 Months of Methadone Maintenance Treatment." *Journal of Addiction Medicine* 5.2 (2011): 141–47. Print.

Pert, C.B., and S.H. Snyder. "Opiate Receptor: Demonstration in Nervous Tissue." *Science* 77 (1973): 1011–14. Web.

Salsitz, Edwin A., Christopher C. Holden, Susan Tross, and Ann Nugent. "Transitioning Stable Methadone Maintenance Patients to Buprenorphine Maintenance." *Journal of Addiction Medicine* 4.2 (2010): 88–91. Print.

Sangi, Sibghatullah, Shahia P. Ahmed, Muhammad Aslam Channa, Muhammad Ashfaq, and Shah Murad Mastoi. *A New and Novel Treatment of Opioid Dependence: Nigella Sativa 500 Mg.* Rep. Ayub Medical College, 2008. Web.

Shiffman, Mitchell L., Fredy Suter, Bruce Bacon, David Nelson, Hugh Harley, Ricard Sola, Stephen D. Shafran, Karl Barange, Amy Lin, Ash Soman, and Stefan Zeuzem. "Peginterferon Alfa-2a and Ribavirin for 16 or 24 Weeks in HCV Genotype 2 or 3." *The New England Journal of Medicine* 357.2 (2007): 124–34. Web.

"Smoking-Attributable Mortality, Years of Potential Life Lost, and Productivity Losses - United States 2000–2004." *Centers for Disease Control and Prevention.* Morbidity and Mortality Weekly Report, 2008. Web.

The National Drug Control Strategy: 1996. The Executive Office of the President of the United States, The White House.

"Treatment of Anxiety Disorders." *National Institute of Mental Health.* Health Topics. Web. <www.nimh.nih.gov>.

United States. Government Accountability Office. *Methadone-associated Overdose Deaths: Factors Contributing to Increased Deaths and Efforts to Prevent Them.* 2009. Print.

U.S. Department of Health and Human Services. *Clinical Guidelines for the Use of Buprenorphine in the Treatment of Opioid Addiction.* U.S. Department of Health and Human Services. Print.

Watkins, K.E., S.B. Hunter, S.L. Wenzel, W. Tu, S.M. Paddock, and P. Ebner. "Prevalence and Characteristics of Clients with Co-occurring Disorders in Outpatient Substance Abuse Treatment." *American Journal of Drug and Alcohol Abuse.* (2004): 749–64. Web.

Wodak, M.D., Alex. "Of Naltrexone." *NSW Users and AIDS Association, Inc.* 2008. Web.

Zimmermann, U., and P. Winklemann. "Withdrawal Phenomena and Dependence Syndrome After the Consumption of Spice Gold" *Deutsches Ärzteblatt International* 106.27 (2009): 464–67. Web.